LOSE IT
FOR THE LAST
TIME

AMY NEWMAN SHAPIRO
RD, CDN, CPT

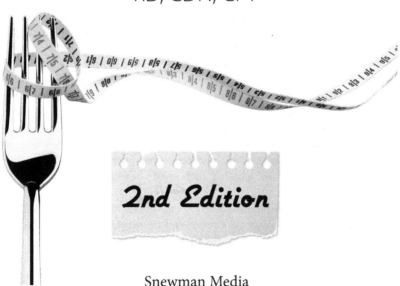

2nd Edition

Snewman Media

The program outlined in this publication is a general guide to better health to be used for educational and informative purposes only. It is not intended as medical advice, diagnosis, or treatment and should not be used in such manner. Before making any changes to your diet or undertaking an exercise program, it is essential that you obtain clearance from your physician. You should always consult with qualified professionals, who can help you by considering your unique circumstances.

The author and publisher shall not be liable to any person or entity with respect to any of the information contained in this book/e-book. The user assumes all risk for any injury, loss, or damage caused or alleged to be caused, directly or indirectly, by using any information described in this program and book.

Although the author and publisher have made every effort to ensure the accuracy of the information contained in this publication at the time of press, the author and publisher do not assume and hereby disclaim any liability to any party for any loss, damage, or disruption caused by errors or omissions, whether such errors or omissions result from negligence, accident, or any other cause.

Mention of specific leaders in research, education, marriage and family therapy, or other authorities in this book does not imply endorsement of this publication.

Internet addresses are accurate at the time of printing.

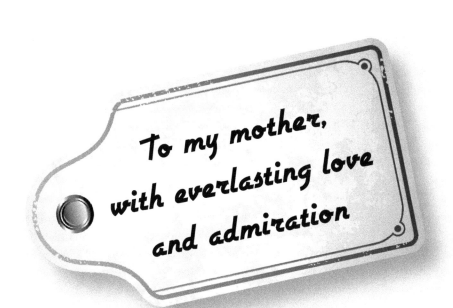

To my mother,
with everlasting love
and admiration

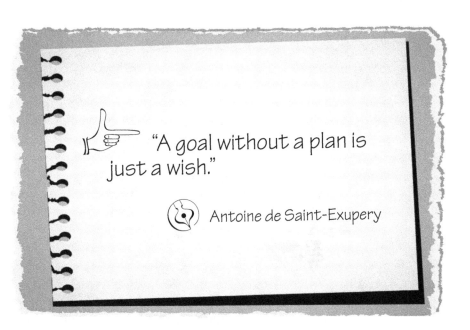

"A goal without a plan is just a wish."

Antoine de Saint-Exupery

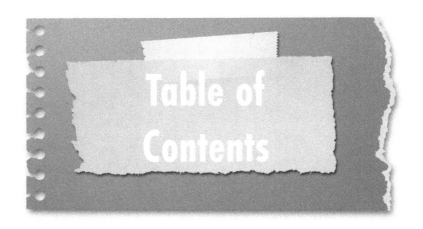

Table of Contents

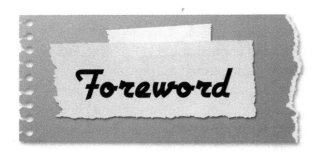

Foreword

Welcome to the Second Edition of *Lose It for the Last Time*. Since the first publication of this book, almost a decade ago, there have been many advancements in the science and technology of weight loss thereby making it easier to access the resources and choose the best fitness monitoring device for your needs. But the tried-and-true weight-loss techniques and skills have mostly remained the same. In this this completely revised and updated edition, I have endeavored to include the latest on scientific breakthroughs and useful technology to help you in your quest to lose weight and get fit—for life.

The idea for writing this book was originally born from a weight loss program I developed for Brookhaven National Laboratories in Upton, NY. As a registered dietitian nutritionist, I was asked to develop and implement a program for weight loss for approximately three thousand employees. I researched many existing programs in the hopes of finding one already developed with a proven track record of results. None of these programs incorporated the specific tools and techniques for behavior change I have used with my clients that have led them to reach their health goals.

The program I first implemented used the LEARN Program for Weight Management by Kelly Brownell as the backbone because the philosophies matched mine, the concepts adhered to the scientific research I trusted, and a priority of the program was to keep records, which was essential for success in my own private practice. I created ten weekly discussions for our group meetings, each one focusing on an idea, concept, or technique for the participants to consider and apply that week. Each successive week built on what had been accomplished the previous weeks.

At every session, the participants were weighed in and monitored to track body composition, blood pressure, blood cholesterol, and blood sugar level for those with diabetes. In addition, changes in quality-of-life ratings were also noted.

The program was an overwhelming success and has evolved over the years to no longer involve the LEARN program. Participants can monitor success by tracking weight loss, and changes in body fat, body mass index, waist and hip circumference, and perceived quality of life. Studies show that weight loss during the ten-week program ranges from a low of ten to sixteen pounds up to thirty-five pounds. Overall, participants succeeded in reducing body fat by an average 6.1 percent. For those whose weight could be tracked long term, 70 percent maintained some or all of their weight loss after one year along with avoiding the weight these participants might have gained if they had not learned new food and lifestyle skills. An additional 20 percent of the participants also came out ahead because even though they regained their lost weight, they didn't put on additional pounds that year.

Hundreds of our participants have improved their eating habits and their relationship with food to lead healthier lifestyles in healthier environments because they also succeeded in bringing these healthy changes to their families, friends, and coworkers. Many even shared with me how their spouse or children began to make improvements to their eating habits and their weight was responding. In fact many people who had been through the program were excited I was writing this book and were happy to contribute their experiences. You will find their stories here to help you see how they applied the techniques and knowledge I was able to offer them and see the difference it made in their lives.

This ten-week program has proven results. Yes, those who did it before you did it under my watchful eye and constant critique and guidance, but I believe you can also experience the same success. All you have to do is apply what I am going to teach you one week at a time. You'll learn to gradually practice your new skills, keep records, and learn from them. My goal is to instruct you to be your own teacher and watchdog, and this will make it possible for you to reach your weight goals.

So, allow yourself a minimum of one week to read, reread, absorb, and implement the concepts in each chapter. Keep in mind this is not a quick fix, magic pill, or promise-the-moon diet, but it is a weight-loss program that works. Remember it took more than a week to gain your excess weight, so it is unrealistic to think you can lose it in a few weeks. Yes there is work for you to do, but your efforts will be rewarded with weight loss you can keep off. I will guide you through each step with the tools and techniques that will make it easy to lose weight and keep it off. By learning new behaviors and making some lifestyle changes you will come to enjoy a lighter, slimmer, and healthier you.

It is essential to remember that your health is your main priority. Sure, most of you are looking to lose weight, but it is paramount (and possible) to be healthy at any weight. Many of the concepts and skills you will be asked to consider and apply are geared to good health. Weight loss will follow.

Acknowledgements

Writing is most often a solitary endeavor. And though the part of my day spent at my computer brings me joy and fulfillment, I would feel disconnected were it not for my cherished friends who stop by for a chat over tea or a glass of wine, call me into the sunshine for a walk through the neighborhood or to hike through a park, and hop on planes to fill my weekend with laughter and adventure.

I am forever grateful to my daughters, for inspiration, for friendship beyond kinship, and whose encouragement to write extends beyond nutrition books. My granddaughters whose wonderment and experimentation refresh my perspective and my creativity. I am privileged to have a mother who has always been my role model, my inspiration, and my constant companion. To my husband Mitch, no words would be enough to thank you for the countless hours you have contributed to IT support, editing, and reassurance. I am so looking forward to where the next chapter of our story takes us.

PJ Dempsey at Log Cabin Editorial has shared my writing journey since the first word of my first book and I am forever grateful for her insights, rewrites, support, and friendship. I so appreciate your tutelage and guidance.

Thank you, Karen Saunders at Karen Saunders & Associates. You, also, have worked with me since my first book. I am grateful that you, the person instrumental in creating a book from my manuscript, is so reliable, responsible, and innovative.

I need also to give a shout out to my dad. Because of him, I honed my skills with words and writing through daily crossword puzzles, weekend scrabble games, assignments to read the classics from the public library and his own prose.

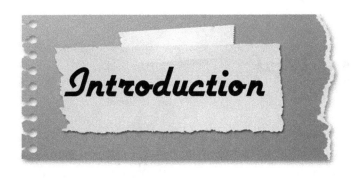

Introduction

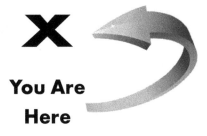

You Are Here

    I remember standing in front of a map in a park trying to orient myself, but I was having difficulty finding the spot marked "X"— You Are Here. That feeling of frustration and impatience hindered my search because I knew I could not move forward until I knew where I stood. Weight loss is much the same in that you need to make that first step in the right direction to put you on the correct path to reach your goal.

    So here is your map to destination weight loss by way of wellness, improved health, weight, and lifestyle changes. By picking up this book you have entered the park and are standing in front of that map with the "X"— You Are Here clearly marked. Congratulations! For some of you, this was a very big step. You may have already looked at other maps or taken other paths to reach your goal. But even though you may have come away having felt like you'd tried and failed, you haven't failed because you are continuing to try. After all, we can only get where we want to be by trying different roads until we find the right one. I can show you the way.

Diets Don't Work

I'm betting that you already know what doesn't work for you, but probably also know what works for you, too. I'll ask you to use those experiences to help you discover and implement new food behaviors and lifestyle habits. If one path leads you to a dead end, we'll figure out how to try another. The bottom line is that it is very important that you discover what is right for your lifestyle. And this is also about change, lasting change. Reaching weight and health goals involve long-term behavior changes. I urge you not to think in terms of "going on a diet". When you "go on a diet" you will inevitably "go off a diet". That translates into returning to the food choices that caused you to gain or re-gain weight before. And, as you know, regained weight is often more than you originally lost.

Change Is Good

You are about to learn how to identify and overcome the food, exercise, and stress behaviors that keep you from reaching your goals along with those you need to discover and incorporate into your current lifestyle. The best part of my program is that, *you* get to decide. Making small changes can lead to big differences when it comes to weight and health. Every step moves you closer toward a specific, measurable, and attainable goal. Never forget that the number you see on the scale is only to be used as a reference. There is no magic number at which you will be transformed into a healthy individual at an ideal weight. Instead, strive to be healthy at any weight. It is easier for a healthy body to lose weight or maintain weight. **Remember, the goal is health, not a number on the scale.**

Choose the Right Path

I am a firm believer in the power of imagery. As a child, I kept myself warm while waiting for the bus by imagining that I was on a sunny warm beach. Likewise, I stay calm through an MRI by reimagining a trip to a favorite place. Imagery is an effective stress management tool that I will be discussing in the book, but I bring it up now because this park with its many paths is a great metaphor for your upcoming endeavor. So I ask to imagine the following: You have entered the park and chosen one path out of many. If you find the one you chose is too steep you might have to choose a longer, less strenuous path that gets you to your destination, slower but with a steady pace. Some paths will lead to discovering new things about yourself that will make it easier to get where you want to be, some will not—but there are lessons to be learned on every path. Remember to always be open to all possibilities. Above all, you need to stay positive when you lose your way and trust that following the map will correct your course to keep you headed towards your goal. But for now, please feel good that you have entered the park. You are here at the beginning of your journey. You are on your way!

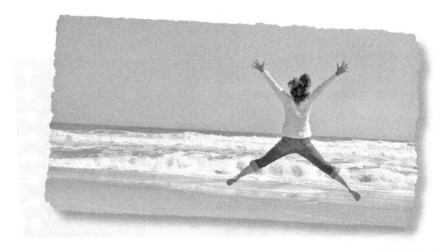

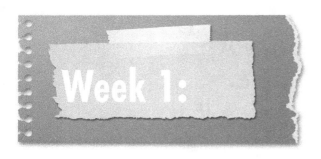

Week 1:

How Did I Get Here?

Our lives are shaped in part by our beliefs. If you believe you are entitled to optimal health and if you believe you can attain your weight and fitness goals, you have a greater chance of success than if you doubt yourself. If you believe you don't have time to exercise, you're not likely to look for exercise options. It's easy to get swept up in our jobs and caring for our families, and use that as an excuse to not eat well or exercise. But think of it in a different way: How much more work might you get done and how much more energy might you have for your kids or your aging parents if you weren't tired all the time—if you were healthier? Think about what is motivating you to lose weight? Surprisingly, fear of getting sick is not a strong motivator, but wanting to play ball with your child is. How about simply wanting to climb the stairs without huffing and puffing? Think of specific motivations like that to help you get through the tough times when weight loss gets challenging.

This brings us to your first exercise.

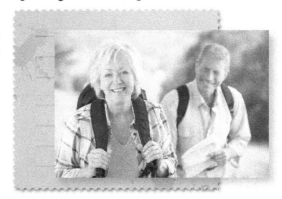

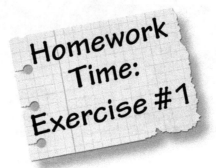

Homework Time: Exercise #1

Write down exactly why you decided to lose weight now.

_____

_____

_____

_____

_____

What is motivating you to succeed?

_____

_____

_____

_____

_____

My Motivation for Change

The most compelling reason I have for making the effort, committing the time and energy, and seeing this through is

I am ready to do what it takes to reach my health goals so that I will be able to

_____

_____

_____

What I will have to give up

_____

_____

_____

_____

_____

_____

_____

How my life will change for the better

_____

_____

_____

_____

_____

_____

_____

At the end of the program I picture myself as

_____

_____

_____

_____

_____

For some, it is quality-of-life issues—having more energy, breathing more easily, for example. For others, it is looking better or feeling better about themselves. However, if you're trying to lose weight because someone else wants you to, stop right now and walk away. Wanting to please others is not enough motivation for the work that lies ahead. If you're still hanging in with me, reread the reasons you wrote down. Are they compelling enough to keep you on track when the going gets tough? If so, let's begin!

So where did your extra weight come from? For most people, the main contributors are our genes (yes, it's true, it's not entirely your fault), our psychological relationship to food, and our environment—both growing up and throughout our lives. But while it's tempting to blame your parents, the truth is that while some people do inherit a tendency to be overweight, genetics alone do not determine what that scale reads. This is because our genes, even though they have the ability to determine how we metabolize fat, carbohydrates, and proteins, are influenced by various internal and external factors that impact how they manifest themselves. These influences also include environmental factors, many of which are within our control, including food intake and lifestyle. You can always change what seems like your destiny. It just might be a little harder than it is for someone who doesn't inherit that tendency.

Think About It

Psychology is a factor in how a person eats because we often use food to soothe us, either as a reward or a punishment. Think of all the celebrating that revolves around food, such as birthday cakes and holiday dinners. Did you get taken out to dinner for bringing home a good report card? Did you get ice cream when you had a cold? These behaviors are formed early on and carry into adulthood, shaping our relationship with food.

For some people, the amount of psychological energy it takes to create change determines how successful they are at losing weight. It takes focus, resolve, patience, and determination to stay the course with a new idea or behavior until permanent change is achieved. That can be compounded by additional circumstances. A person with disordered eating has emotional barriers to work through. The person concerned about a financial situation may have less mental focus on the tasks involved in weight loss. All this affects your focus.

Change What You Can, Accept What You Can't

Your personal environment is the largest contributing factor in how much you weigh. The social climate in which you live, your ethnic background, how you celebrate, the availability of food throughout the day, and enticements at the mall, the gas station, or even your own kitchen determine what you eat, when you eat, and how much you eat.

Rarely does knowing the cause of overweight actually help you lose weight. However, consider it in the context of change. There are things we can change and things we cannot. For example, you cannot change the past. If you were raised with food as a reward or to soothe tough times, you can't change that. For many people the cookie they got with a Band-Aid after they skinned a knee morphs into an ice cream sundae after a hard day at work as an adult. But we can change the food choices in our homes and the behaviors that affect what and how much we eat as well as how we use food for comfort and reward. These are lifestyle changes that help you lose weight.[1]

Why Diets Don't Work

The reason most weight-loss diets don't work is that they focus on limiting or eliminating specific foods or entire food groups, like carbs for instance. This removes an important source of fuel for the body, along with vitamins, minerals and antioxidants important for optimal health. The diet also eliminates the foods from your daily intake that you may tend to overeat, such as pasta, cereal, or chips. But such an approach does not maintain long-term weight loss and weight maintenance.[2] Here's why:

Cutting out carbohydrates means you successfully eliminate some calories, so you lose weight. In some cases, that weight is from a good deal of water loss, which—darn it—always returns. Still, because your weight is heading in the right direction—down—you feel successful. But once you've lost the weight and if you resume your old eating patterns, lo and behold, the pounds will return and often more than you lost. If you're like many dieters, you will probably diet again—and the yo-yo cycling of weight begins.

The problem with this all-too-familiar scenario is that you're not making the long-term changes in how you behave around food to sustain weight loss or to maintain your new lower weight. It doesn't take a rocket scientist to figure out that if you return to your usual way of eating you will continue to pack on the pounds. In addition, weight loss causes the body to produce appetite-stimulating hormones. Think about it. The brain cannot differentiate between starvation and a self-imposed calorie deficit. Therefore it goes into self-preservation mode by sending signals to all body systems to eat and store energy. In real life this amounts to dieting actually setting you up to regain the weight.

Is there anything good about diets? Yes. What works is the structure diets bring to eating. A diet provides a plan. It's this manipulation of food intake and the lowering of calories that effectively leads to weight loss. This "diet" mentality, however, does not lead to long-term success. A chronic dieter relies on willpower and rule following as tools for success, so when the scale starts creeping back up dieters often blame it on their lack of willpower and fortitude when the real problem is not changing the behaviors that could prevent weight gain.

What we eat is based on many things: food likes and dislikes, what's available, what's convenient, and lifestyle. Those are all very individual. So why should—or could—anyone else tell us what to eat and what not to eat? Moreover, diets make you feel deprived which often results in cravings and binging. And diets that label certain foods as "forbidden" can make you feel like you've failed if you "cheat" and eat those foods even just once. But, rest assured, 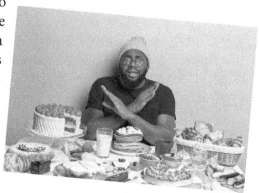 one fall off the wagon does not a fallen dieter make.

Diets are also counterproductive in other ways. Diets cause atrophy of our internal cues that tell us when to eat and when to stop. Diets can increase stress and fatigue because of feelings of deprivation and the lack of sufficient calories and nutrients. Quick weight loss actually triggers the release of brain chemicals to fight to replace fat stores and restore weight. Severe calorie restriction slows metabolism. Weight loss also increases production of appetite hormones tending to increase calorie intake and restore lost weight.

Quick (and Temporary) vs. Steady (and Permanent)

The weight-loss method I offer here is not about a quick fix. Permanent weight loss occurs when you make lasting lifestyle and attitude changes without restriction or deprivation. Nutrition affects your mood, emotional state, energy level, and health. Weight loss is easier when you are healthy, but optimal nutrition rarely exists with a diet that deprives the body of a food group or appropriate calories.[3] Permanent weight loss can only be achieved when lasting lifestyle change occurs. Small changes in your food intake or physical activity can make a big difference.

Your long-term goal may be loss of weight but be realistic. It may have taken months or years to put those pounds on and expecting to lose them all in a flash will only set you up for failure. This will only make you feel negative about yourself and your efforts. So you need to be realistic about setting your initial weight goal. The healthiest weight loss is gradual, just one to two pounds per week. For someone who is very overweight or obese, a weight loss of 10 percent in three months is a realistic goal. Remember, this is not a race. As long as the weight is coming off even losing half a pound is significant because it means the behaviors you have changed are working. Being realistic about how much you can lose also lessens the chances of you being disappointment in your progress. Negative thoughts only get in the way of success.

Short-term efforts are the small changes that lead to permanent weight loss. The hard part is making changes consistently so that they eventually become healthy habits you don't have to think about. Establishing a new habit takes thought, planning, and practice. Yet a new behavior can become a habit as fast as in three weeks if done consistently. Once a new habit becomes part of your everyday experience, a lifestyle change has occurred.

Everyday goals must be realistic to be achievable. If walking the dog leaves you breathless then your chances of running a marathon are unattainable in the near-term. If you have five children to get ready for school then going to the gym before 8 a.m. may not be doable. If you really enjoy munching on chips then vowing to never eat chips again may be unrealistic. Everyday goals also need to be measurable. For example, a goal of including one cup of vegetables every night at dinner instead of simply vowing to eat more vegetables increases the odds of successfully following through. Also consider wearing a pedometer, Fitbit, or smart watch and walking 10,000 steps a day as a measurable exercise goal, instead of just guessing. Maintaining normalized blood sugar and blood pressure levels are also measurable, achievable, and potentially lifesaving goals. All too often, success—or the lack of it— is determined by a number on the scale. But your weight is affected

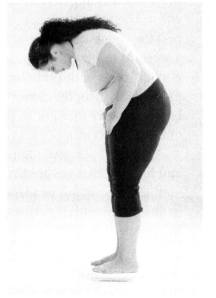

by a number of factors, including fluid retention, salt-intake, and hormone shifts. Remember, too, that increased physical activity increases muscle mass and metabolism. The extra muscle increases metabolism and aids weight loss in the long term. However, be aware that there may be no initial change in weight and the increased muscle may even show a weight gain. This is normal because building muscle results in microtears in the fibers which cause temporary inflammation and water retention. Also, the body provides energy to those muscles in the form of glycogen and it increases stored glycogen when you exercise regularly. Glycogen requires water to fuel muscles showing up as a weight gain from water retention. The good news is that as your muscles acclimate to regular exercise the extra water is released and the extra weight is lost. Moreover, the number on the scale cannot measure success such as health gains like less body fat or lower blood pressure.

So, to weigh or not to weigh? The choice is yours. For some people, positive results on the scale help them stay focused on their new behaviors and goals. Others find weighing in discouraging, because the ups and downs on the scale may be unrelated to behavior changes. And negative thoughts can lead to negative effort. For them, the scale is not useful. Determine what works best for you, but I encourage you to weigh yourself at least once a week to assess progress. In addition, although not highly accurate, scales with body fat analyzers may help you assess improvement in body composition. Or consider an easy-to-use blood pressure monitor to provide you with a different measure of health success.

Assessing, acknowledging, and rewarding positive behavior and lifestyle changes are the sure way to get results. This means you need a method of identifying the behaviors you may need to change. Identifying daily and weekly goals and changing your behaviors to meet those goals will give you a way to measure your accomplishments (or get back on track if what you are doing isn't working). This may be time consuming at first but keeping records will prove to be an invaluable tool as you progress.

You Must Know Where You've Been To Know Your Next Steps

Start by taking a look at where you are right now, nutritionally speaking, by starting a food and activity journal.

Research has found that journaling leads to greater weight loss success. Keeping a journal will keep you on track, help identify barriers to weight loss in your daily intake, hold you accountable, record progress, and keep you goal oriented. People who keep records succeed more than people who don't. A study done by Kaiser Permanente of about 1,700 people found that out of the two-thirds of participants who experienced weight loss, those keeping food diaries lost twice as much weight as those who didn't do so. Simply put, a food and exercise journal/diary keeps you honest. You exercise because you know you will have to write it down. You may skip that cookie if you know you have to record eating it. Keeping records affects commitment, shows progress, and provides feedback. It may not be fun, but it is important.

A food journal will also help you identify current habits, food intake, calorie intake, when you eat, and how much you eat. A journal helps to improve eating patterns and increase control over what you eat and how much. It is not necessarily WHAT you are eating, but WHEN and HOW MUCH that may make the difference.

If you want to go old-school with pen and paper, then use the following template for your food and activity journal. It will take more time to calculate calorie intake from food labels and other sources, but it will be much easier to accomplish this feat if you are technologically challenged.

Food Journal

TIME	FOOD EATEN	AMOUNT	CALORIES

Activity Log

TIME	ACTIVITY	MINUTES	STEPS

There are also several easily accessible food journal options available on various websites and smart phone apps that provide databases of food and nutritional information to help with tracking portion size and calories, in addition to carbohydrate, protein, and fat intake. The most popular are www.myfitnesspal.com, www.loseit.com, and www.mynetdiary.com. It is important that you find the method that is easiest for you to use so you will be more likely to consistently monitor food and meal choices and adjust where necessary to meet your goals.

For the first week, record everything that you eat and drink, the time of day, exactly what you put in your mouth and how much. (You may refer to the chart above to create your own food and activity journal or download a free PDF of the food and activity journal at www.LoseItfortheLastTime.com.) Do not skip this step. It's *the* most important exercise you will do. Get out the measuring cups, measuring spoons, and scale. For example, at 7:00 a.m. pour your usual amount of cold cereal into a bowl, then pour it into a measuring cup to know exactly how much you're eating. Next, pour the milk into a measuring cup before adding it to the cereal, increase the amount, if necessary. Record EVERY detail, including the time you eat and the type of cereal and milk. Sometimes you may need to refer to the package information. Or, when you are splitting a half-pound of chicken into two servings, then one serving will be four ounces.

When eating out, you'll have to rely on making an educated guess. Below are some handy guidelines to help you visually size up your meal:

- ▶ *3 ounces protein = palm of your hand*
- ▶ *1/2 cup pasta or cooked vegetables = a cupped hand*
- ▶ *1 cup salad = 2 cupped hands*
- ▶ *1 teaspoon sauce or dressing = tip of your thumb to the first knuckle*

- ▶ *1 ounce of cheese = length and width of your thumb*
- ▶ *1 cup of cereal = your fist*
- ▶ *1 serving of fruit = your fist*

Two crucial credos to follow:

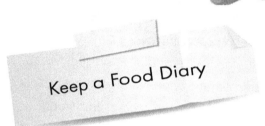

Keep a Food Diary

Don't assume you know how much you're eating, no matter how many diets you've followed in the past. Everyone tends to underestimate how much they eat. Immediately after eating, record what you eat so you don't forget or remember it incorrectly.

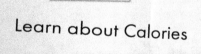

Learn about Calories

Calories determine weight. When calories in equals calories out weight stays the same—a simple equation, often ignored. It's not the amount of carbohydrates or fat you ingest per se, but the total number of calories you eat and how many of them you burn off through physical activity. Calorie counting is not the focus here and certainly not a lifestyle change, but it is a helpful learning tool. I'm not going to reinvent the wheel by listing calories because many resources already provide that information. I recommend checking out www.fooducate.com, www.fitday.com, and www.sparkpeople.com, for calorie and nutrition facts. If you are using the non-digital paper method, get a copy of the calorie guide published by Calorie King.

> Recording the times of day you eat and how much you eat is also a critical step for identifying eating patterns. I recommend recording every time you eat, this includes meals and all snacking. Most online and smart phone tools have a notes section where you can record additional information.

Learn What Triggers Your Eating

The first weekly goal concerns learning about your eating habits: what foods you like, how much you typically eat, your pattern of meals and snacks, situations in which you tend to overeat, meals you often skip, emotions and social situations that trigger your eating.

In essence, your goal is to become aware of all the factors that are keeping you from losing weight. During the week, analyze your food journal for clues as to what behaviors may be problematic. Look for small changes you can make in how you eat now that may help you shed pounds.

You also have to learn about when your calorie intake is high. For example, maybe you're taking in too many calories at night. If so, one solution would be to eat breakfast every day if you haven't been doing so regularly. Look at your snack habits: Are your snacks typically high in sugar, fat—or both? Pay particular attention to any emotional eating you can identify, including the foods you eat when stressed, lonely, celebrating, depressed, or bored. Emotional eating is often situational, cyclical, and habitual, which makes it a tough habit to break and may require a great deal of psychological energy and, therefore, may slow your weight loss. If you suspect being an emotional eater then consider consulting a behavioral health specialist.

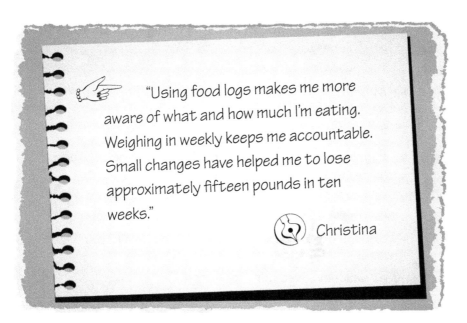

"Using food logs makes me more aware of what and how much I'm eating. Weighing in weekly keeps me accountable. Small changes have helped me to lose approximately fifteen pounds in ten weeks."

Christina

Eliminate One Easy-To-Do-Without Food

Your goal for the week is to evaluate your food diary to determine where you're getting those extra calories and then to choose one of those sources and eliminate it. Choose something you will not miss and find an adequate lower-calorie substitute. Don't forget that even one important change can reap big benefits. Here are some ideas to get you thinking, along with what you'll gain from subtracting (a better profile in the mirror!):

- ▶ *Flavored seltzer/unsweetened iced tea instead of regular soda (1 12-oz soft drink per day):*
  - ▷ Calories saved per year = 51,100
  - ▷ Pounds lost per year = 14.5

- ▶ *Fruit preserve instead of butter on a bagel (3 per week):*
  - ▷ Calories saved per year = 14,976
  - ▷ Pounds lost per year = 4

- ▶ *Mustard on a sandwich instead of mayo (3 per week):*
  - ▷ Calories saved per year = 13,260
  - ▷ Pounds lost per year = 4

- ▶ *Egg white omelet instead of a whole egg omelet (2 eggs twice/week):*
  - ▷ Calories saved per year = 12,272
  - ▷ Pounds lost per year = 3.5

- ▶ *Skip the cheese on sandwiches and burgers (2 per week):*
  - ▷ Calories saved per year = 10,400
  - ▷ Pounds lost per year = 3

Step on It—
Walk Your Way To Fitness

Eliminating foods you can live without is easy and rewarding because you magically take in fewer calories without feeling deprived, but that only goes so far. As I mentioned earlier, a lifestyle that leads to weight loss and supports weight maintenance must also include physical activity.[4,5] Exercising does not require a gym membership or fancy home equipment, although both are certainly nice to have. Instead, consider that you already have a ready-made gym with exercise equipment right in your very own home or office, including the fact that you also have exercise equipment attached to your body. Intrigued? Well believe it or not you can lose weight just by walking more—no special

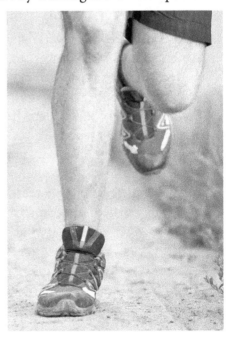

equipment required. Let's start with simple walking, what I call the first category of walking for your first-week goal of establishing a baseline for your physical activity.

Walking is a simple and effective mode of exercising which requires no special equipment or a gym, but a pedometer or a fitness tracker like Fitbit or an Apple watch makes it easier to keep track of daily steps and progress. For a simple, but highly accurate, method look for a pedometer that counts steps (either with or without miles). However, if you already use more sophisticated technology, they are extremely useful despite their reported inaccuracies. Wear your activity counting device of choice every day and take it off when you go to bed so you have an accurate record of the number of steps you take.

You do not need to invest in anything fancy, however, upgrades like an appealing feature on some pedometers is the ability to distinguish between aerobic and non-aerobic walking, may appeal to some people. It may also help if your device can record and graph your progress on the computer. Another popular feature is the ability to calculate the number of calories burned.

Fitness trackers do more than calculate how far you've walked; they also keep track of all the exercise you get from the "activities of daily living" (ADLs). This daily exertion comprises all your normal daily activities that burn calories without you thinking about it—but these burned calories count, too.

A second category of walking involves raising your heart rate which not only strengthens the heart but also burns calories. Keep in mind that several short bouts of exercise have health benefits as potent as longer sessions.

For this week, wear your activity tracker all day, every day, and record the number of steps you get from both planned exercise activity and any added steps from your ADLs. I recommend recording this in a separate activity journal and not directly entering this information into an app/website which tends to increase suggested calorie goals when exercise is added. This is because many people use this as a reason to eat more since more calories are being burned, impeding weight loss. Remember, weight loss happens when you burn more calories than you eat, the calorie deficit is what causes weight loss.

So what's the plan?

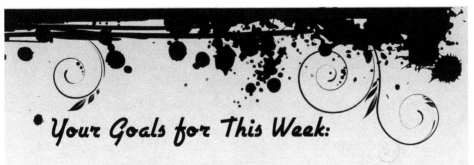

Your Goals for This Week:

1. Use a daily food journal to record what time you eat or drink anything, what it is you consumed, the amount, and the calories.

2. Choose a digital food journal or refer to the samples on page 12 and 13 to create your own, downloadable pdfs are available at https://loseitforthelasttime.com/index.php/food-journal/.

    a. *Look at what your food choices are, how much you eat, the time of day you eat, and what you are not eating enough of*

    b. *Become aware of changes you can make that may lead to weight loss*

    c. *Choose at least one source of calories in your current intake that you can reduce or eliminate*

3. Get an activity tracker (Omron Alvita Pedometer, Fitbit, Garmin, Samsung Galaxy, Apple Watch)

    a. *Record the number of steps you take each day both from your normal daily routine and planned exercise*

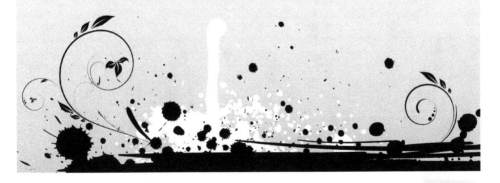

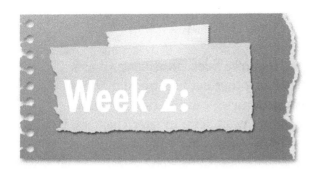

Week 2:

Change Will Happen Inside Out

Your completed daily food journal and activity log are your measures of success for the past week. Sure, it's wonderful if the scale reflects your effort to eliminate or reduce a calorie source, but don't panic if the same number is staring up at you when you weigh yourself. Instead, congratulate yourself for completing the goals laid out in the first week and vow to continue your commitment to make behavior and lifestyle changes. You should also not lose sight of the fact that you now have a clearer understanding of what, when, and how much you eat because you learned to red-flag in your journal the times of the day or particular food choices where change could lead to weight loss.

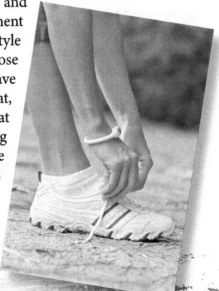

More kudos are also due if you've been measuring your activity level with a pedometer or other activity tracker. Studies show that simply wearing a pedometer can increase how much you walk in a day.[6] It's all about awareness. In later chapters, I will introduce additional ways to refine your calorie intake and physical activity level.

Metabolic Mumbo Jumbo

So, why can't you lose weight? The system is rigged against us. The biological interaction of genes (inherited traits), hormones, and brain chemicals that regulate appetite and fat storage direct the brain as to what, when, and how much to eat. Unfortunately, this system is designed to keep the body alive when no food is available and that means storing unused calories as fat—not eliminating them. Eating more calories than we burn packs on the pounds. Restrictive diets do manage to eliminate eating extra calories, but reducing food intake causes the brain to react by decreasing metabolism (the rate at which the body burns calories for energy) thereby preserving calories.

These real physical and physiological factors challenge losing weight as an attempt at self-preservation. The body fights to maintain weight just as it does to sustain body temperature. This is why quickly losing weight triggers the brain to replace lost fat stores and restore any lost pounds because it cannot differentiate between intentional weight loss and starvation. Simply put, all weight loss triggers an increase in appetite hormones resulting in increased hunger when you eat less. Therefore, successful weight loss can only happen if you learn to adjust what you eat and outsmart biology by improving metabolism by increasing physical activity (this will be motivation to increase your step goal) and altering what you choose to eat for meals and snacks and when you eat them—timing.

Increasing physical activity is self-explanatory, but altering meal time can be counterintuitive as long intervals without eating actually signal starvation to the brain. This causes metabolism to slow to conserve calories by slowing the rate at which they burn off. This "starvation mechanism" also boosts the body's tendency to store fat. So don't think you're doing yourself a favor when you skip breakfast or lunch because the body will only crave larger portions of food later on to satisfy your level of hunger. To make matters worse, the body will then store the calories you don't need for immediate energy as fat in anticipation of the next period of starvation. This is why skipping meals is always counterproductive if you're trying to lose weight.

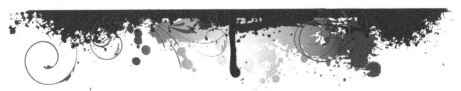

Blame It on Your Parents

Much of the way we view food comes from childhood, family food behaviors, and ethnic and religious cultures. Childhood experiences shape how we use food, either as a reward, to celebrate, or to soothe. Changing the way you view food will help you to reduce your food intake. For instance, try choosing a non-food reward the next time you want to treat yourself. Instead of dinner out or an ice cream sundae, treat yourself to a movie or a massage. One woman told me that she put a dollar in reserve every day she reached her activity goal and then used that money to treat herself to a visit at a ritzy hair salon she had always wanted to try. Another said she used the money toward a trip to Disney World.

Celebrations and holidays each present a minefield of opportunities to overeat. Most cultures celebrate with large amounts of foods and delicacies for religious holidays, weddings, and rites of passage. Add to that Thanksgiving feasts, Memorial Day picnics, and all the holidays in between, plus birthdays, and you average 2.4 occasions each month in which to overindulge. This is why my program is designed to show you ways to change the way you handle such situations. Your biggest hurdle will change from overeating to getting your family and friends to accept your new attitude at food-centered events.

One childhood experience many of us share is guilt over wasting food. If, like me, you were raised to feel bad any time food was wasted because you were told that there were people starving somewhere, I suggest you contribute what you can to help stop hunger in the world and in your community, but the abundance of food in many of our lives has made food detrimental to our health. So let go of the notion instilled in us long ago. Cancel your membership to the clean-your-plate club right now. It is okay, in fact it is imperative, that you stop eating all the food put in front of you just because you were served it or because you paid for it. This doesn't mean it needs to go to waste either. Leftovers from dinner can be repurposed as lunch the next day or perhaps even another dinner. This can even help cut down on meal preparation and cost if you get two meals out of one.

What's Sleep Got to Do with It?

Another factor to consider in the struggle with weight is the amount of sleep you get. Poor sleep quality can be caused by sleep apnea, an infant, a snoring partner, stress, or menopause. Poor quality of sleep creates stress impacting both brain and body function. Any decrease in mental energy and the lack of focus it brings can be detrimental when trying to lose or maintain weight. The stress brought on by fatigue also causes metabolic hormonal changes that increase blood sugar and fat storage.

The stress brought on by a lack of sleep also impacts the hormones controlling hunger and fullness. Not enough sleep increases the production of ghrelin, a hormone that increases hunger.

Yes, not getting enough sleep also makes you hungry. What's more, being sleep-impaired not only makes you eat more, but it also leads you to make poor food decisions. We have evidence linking high-fat diets to insomnia, proof that sleep affects food choices and food habits affect sleep. When we don't get enough sleep, we also choose to eat more fat. Researchers also found that people who slept less than seven hours ate more carbohydrates and less protein, a sign of a brain short on energy seeking out its preferred form of fuel. Furthermore, a low protein intake (less than 19% of total calories) led to difficulty in falling asleep as well as poor sleep quality. Caffeine and alcohol intake should also be monitored as to not only how much, but also what time of day it's consumed as that also determines its impact on sleep.

If you're having trouble sleeping, download a yoga or meditation app, listen to calming music, drink chamomile tea, or take magnesium or melatonin supplements. Make sure the room temperature is conducive to sleep (68 F. is ideal for most people). You may also need to change your evening routine and get to sleep earlier. Eliminate the blue light emitted from televisions and personal devices that are known to interfere with sleep quality. Most electronic devices have a setting to block blue light and eyeglasses can also be ordered with a blue light filter. If your problem is sleep apnea or snoring, go to a sleep clinic for a sleep study. Sleep apnea not only contributes to being overweight but is also a factor in heart disease. Explore your options as there are several noninvasive treatments available. (One client began using a CPAP machine for apnea and lost twenty pounds in the first five weeks.) If it's your partner's snoring that is keeping you awake, try ear plugs or a white noise machine to muffle the sound.

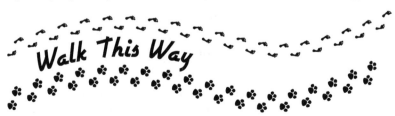

Walk This Way

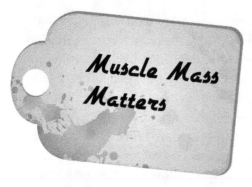

Muscle Mass Matters

Many people blame weight gain on age or menopause, but the fact is metabolism changes very little between the ages of 20-60, unless influenced by behavioral changes. After age 60, however, metabolism decreases about seven percent per decade, a difference of about 100-200 calories a day every ten years. Actually, weight gain as you age is often a result of the change in your activity level. Less activity causes you to burn fewer calories and fosters a loss of muscle mass; both contribute to middle-age weight gain. The good news is that both can be prevented with regular exercise.

When it comes to menopause, you're adding a major change in hormone levels, fatigue from disrupted sleep and sometimes extra stress, which might lead to eating as a coping mechanism. Moreover, women experience a shift in fat storage during menopause that may occur irrespective of whether they are overweight. A woman's body is designed to store fat around the hips and thighs to support pregnancy. At menopause, the drop in sex-specific hormones causes a shift of fat stores to the abdomen, more closely resembling where men carry extra fat. This is why women experience a thickening at the waist. This abdominal fat increases the risk of heart disease and may be the reason why postmenopausal women are at greater risk of heart disease. Maintaining a healthy weight and activity level can reduce the development of abdominal fat.

Our sedentary lifestyles have led to weight gain. Modern technology has decreased our opportunity to move. If you live in a city and can walk to work, to school, and on errands, you are at an advantage. Those of us who live in suburban or rural areas rely on cars or public transportation. Even bicycling as a way to get around is often impractical because of the congestion of cars on pedestrian unfriendly roads. Think of all the conveniences that have developed that have reduced movement even in our own homes. For example, remote controls, portable phones, dishwashers, and clothes dryers. What about at work? Office workers gained weight with the advent of e-mail because they no longer had to walk to deliver paper memos. Today, many of us spend most of every day glued to a chair facing a computer or using another electronic device our only "exercise" consisting of keystrokes and electronic buttons. The truth is that to maintain weight you must burn as many calories as you eat and to lose weight you need to burn more calories than you eat. Knowing how

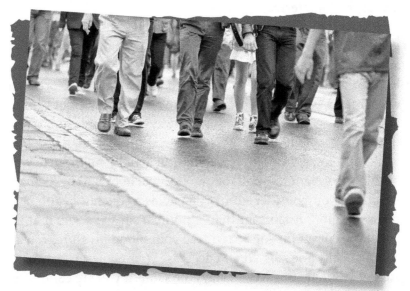

much physical activity it takes to burn calories in specific foods will help you make good food choices. Known as exercise equivalents, they are based on body weight and exercise duration and intensity. Consider a Taco Bell Beef Taco Salad (760 calorie) has an exercise equivalent that requires a 170-pound person to climb stairs for 1 hour 15 minutes to prevent storing those calories as fat. Exercise equivalent calculators are available at *University of Rochester Medical Center:* https://www.urmc.rochester.edu/en

cyclopedia/content.aspx?ContentTypeID=41&ContentID=Cal orieBurnCalc and *American Council on Exercise:* https://www. acefitness.org/resources/everyone/tools-calculators/physical-activity-calorie-counter/

We have already examined compelling reasons why exercise is important. Let's consider the health benefits of physical activity beyond body weight. Exercise improves physical and emotional well-being. It lowers cholesterol and blood sugar levels and reduces blood pressure. Aerobic exercise increases endorphins, those feel-good brain chemicals. It increases positive feelings about ourselves because we feel virtuous, empowered. Best of all, exercise is the best predictor of keeping weight off for the long term.

Always remember that increasing physical activity also increases muscle mass that in turn improves body composition and overall health. The resulting increase in metabolism also leads to long-term weight loss but be aware that the short-term effect is excess fluid retention that can register as weight gain on a scale. This is why the scale is not always a true indicator of fat- or weight-loss failure or success.

Bottom line? If you increase physical activity to improve your health, the weight loss will follow. The goal here is to be fit at any weight. If you consider all of your goals, reducing health concerns are more important than a number on the scale. If at the end of this program you've reduced your blood pressure, you are automatically a success. If you decrease your cholesterol, you're a success. Even if your weight stays the same, if you are committed

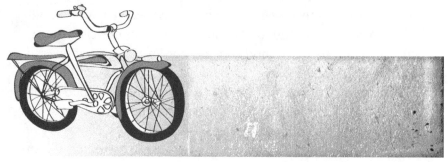

> "I went from 42.6 percent body fat to 32.8 percent body fat, so basically dropped 10 percent of my body fat! I had had my cholesterol checked a year ago and it was 205. Recently, I had the opportunity to get my cholesterol checked again and after approximately two months of eating healthier and exercising, my cholesterol was down to 128."
>
> Sarah

and performing daily physical activity, you are a success. Keep in mind, exercise doesn't have to be strenuous or take up a big chunk of your day. Even small amounts count, and they add up. Most of our daily movements are for activities of daily living (ADLs). James A. Levine, MD, PhD, coined the phrase "non-exercise activity thermogenesis."[7] Both phrases refer to the calories burned through movement that's not a planned activity. By forgoing some modern conveniences, you can increase your activity level, burn more calories, and improve your health—all by just going about your everyday business. It's not hard; you just have to think about it. Here are some suggestions to start:

▶ Park your car farther away from stores when running errands.

▶ Carry groceries into the house one bag at a time.

▶ Mow the lawn. Rake leaves.

▶ Mop the floors. Vacuum the rugs.

▶ Pace when talking on the phone.

> ► *Find and use the stairs instead of taking the elevator a floor or two (it's also faster).*

> ► *Walk the dog at least twice daily (it's good for you both!)*

One of my clients began getting off the subway one stop before her office, then walking the rest of the way. This later led her to do the same thing on her way home.

The key is to find whatever excuse you can to add steps to your day. And that activity tracker you've been wearing is going to keep tract of those additional steps for you. You have your baseline from last week; now you're going to watch that number rise.

The American Heart Association recommends 10,000 steps each day for heart health and weight maintenance. Set reasonable step goals to get closer and closer to that 10K number per day. If you were at 3,000 steps last week, aim for 4,000 this week. It's not a race, it's a challenge to simply keep improving. If you record your steps each day, it will motivate you.

But don't stop there. Consider the calorie-burning, gut-busting, heart-strengthening results you get from brisk aerobic walking. Again, don't be concerned about the length of time you can com-

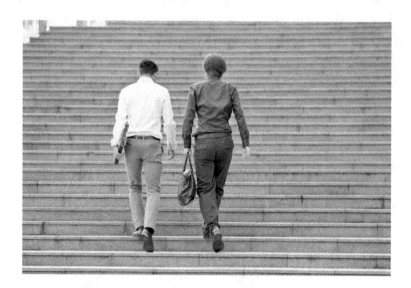

fortably walk or the pace just yet. Start from wherever you are right now. The important thing is establishing exercise as part of your lifestyle. Right now all you need to do or be concerned about is yourself and how and when you are going to get the job done.

A great way to assess aerobic walking is to use the talk test. If you can hold a conversation or recite the alphabet without getting breathy, chances are you are walking too slow to have much of an effect on your health. If you are breathing heavily, you are exerting yourself too much. When walking at an aerobic pace, you need to take a breath every three to five words and are exercising at an appropriate intensity. When possible, extend how long you exercise. Also consider changing your routine so you don't get bored if you have been doing the same thing for a long time. Besides it will renew your interest and commitment and a new exercise or routine may challenge new muscle groups and add to total calories burned. Whatever your starting point, it's time to get moving.

Quite often, people say they don't have time to exercise. That's an excuse, not an obstacle. Wear that pedometer while you walk around the block or on the treadmill. Every step counts. Short bouts of aerobic exercise count. No time at work? Spend your mid-morning and mid-afternoon break climbing the stairs or take a brisk walk before lunch. At your child's baseball practice, bring your sneakers and walk around the field while you watch. Are you on the couch every night watching TV? Find room for a piece of exercise equipment in front of the TV. When I need an extra incentive to use my stationary bike, I reward myself by watching a streaming series I have been wanting to see, but the rule is that I can only watch it while pedaling. The more suspenseful the series, the greater the incentive to get on my bike.

Banish any negative thoughts you have about exercise. Instead, think about your walks and workouts in terms of a relaxing distraction and a way to blow off stress, or playtime, instead of exercise. This will not only make the time spent exercising as something to look forward to, but also as a positive influence on your eating afterward. If you think of a physical activity session purely as exercise you are more likely to be tired and ill-tempered after. You are also more likely to load up on calories, particularly comfort foods, like sugar, as a reward than if you thought of this activity as a pleasurable one. Some suggestions for making exercise a more fun experience include listening to music or podcasts, taking your activity outdoors to enjoy the fresh air and scenery, or inviting a friend or family member to join you and making it a time to socialize. When exercise is fun you won't feel the need to reward yourself with foods or unhealthy snacks. But, if, in spite of your best efforts, exercise is still a chore that you need to reward yourself for doing, then seek out a healthier way to treat yourself that doesn't include eating.

So, When Do We Eat?

Review your daily food journal beginning from week one. Take note of whether you are eating three meals a day or are routinely skipping meals. Make a note of which meals you are skipping and read on for suggestions on how to eat regularly without adding calories.

Breakfast is a meal often forgotten. Think about it. You don't expect your car to get you to work or school without gas, but you expect your body—also a machine— to run without fuel. And don't say you're too busy to stop and eat lunch. The consequences are not worth it.

Remember how metabolism slows down when you go hungry and the amount of food it takes to fill that empty feeling hunger creates. Consider, too, how fast you eat when that hungry. It takes your stomach twenty minutes to tell your brain it's had enough. So if you are very hungry and eating fast, chances are

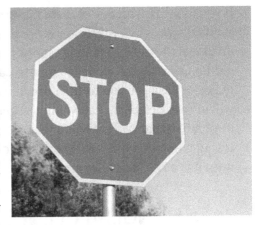

you are not stopping when you have eaten enough to satisfy that hunger and have probably overeaten if you stopped after feeling very full. The human body is programmed to experience some level of hunger if meals are spaced more than four hours apart.

If your meals are more than four hours apart, then it is appropriate to snack. That snack should provide between 50 to 150 calories, which is enough to fuel the body and brain, reduce immediate hunger, and help control hunger at the next meal. Another benefit is that snacking will enable you to cut back on how much you eat at the next meal. You may actually need to eat more often to consume fewer calories. In essence, snacking between meals can cut calories. Healthy snacking provides fuel and nutrients when energy is low or other signs of hunger are evident.

In your food log, take note of the times of day you eat. Are you only eating when you're hungry? Consider these two scenarios:

► *You have breakfast at 8:00 a.m. and lunchtime is at noon, but at the 10:00 a.m. meeting bagels are served and you eat one smeared with butter even though you aren't hungry.*

► *At lunch you eat everything you packed or were served because it is there or because you don't want to feel hungry later that day.*

If you identify with one of these patterns, then plan to have snacks available for when meals are more than four hours apart, so you don't feel the need to tank up at one meal while anticipating hunger before it's even close to time to eat the next one. Doing this makes it easy for you to turn down food because you know you will always be able to eat when you get hungry again. In fact, it is imperative that you eat when you are hungry and are able to stop eating when you are not. The first tool you are to work on, then, until it is a new behavior and a habit, is the hunger/fullness scale.

HUNGER/FULLNESS SCALE

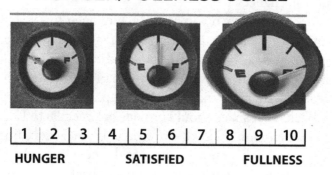

| 1 | 2 | 3 | 4 | 5 | 6 | 7 | 8 | 9 | 10 |

HUNGER   **SATISFIED**   **FULLNESS**

On a scale of one to ten, with one being that you feel as hungry as you'd be if you haven't eaten in days and ten being you feel as full as if you just finished Thanksgiving dinner, your ideal number should always be about a five. If, instead you are at a three, then you are ready for a meal or a snack. If you wait until hunger makes you unfocused, gives you a headache, or makes you cranky, then you are letting yourself get too hungry. If you do this too many times and ignore the rumbling in your tummy or the drop in your energy level, you can get to the point where you no longer recognize the hunger cues your brain is sending. If this happens, you must start paying attention to your hunger cues or follow an eating schedule so the awareness of the cues will return. Don't eat by the clock permanently, but it may be necessary at first, until your ability to recognize hunger cues returns.

Now, here is the real challenge: You need to stop eating when you are no longer hungry. When you are a five on the hunger/fullness scale, your stomach is satisfied (notice I said stomach, not necessarily your mouth and taste buds). Any calories you eat past the point of satiety are not needed by your body, and will be stored as fat.

So, if you overeat at dinner and then park yourself on the couch for a night in front of the TV, the only thing your body can do with those extra calories is to store them because none are being burned off. If you've compounded the problem by skipping a meal or not snacking between lunch and dinner, then your body is primed to being even more efficient at storing those extra calories. This results in weight gain. From now on, always assess your hunger on the hunger/fullness scale and eat when you are a three and stop eating when you are a five.

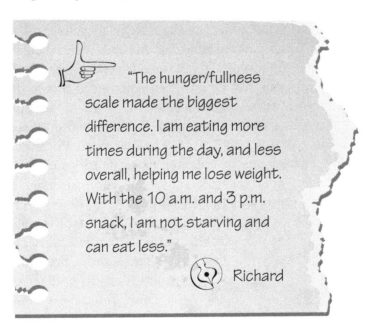

"The hunger/fullness scale made the biggest difference. I am eating more times during the day, and less overall, helping me lose weight. With the 10 a.m. and 3 p.m. snack, I am not starving and can eat less."

Richard

Be careful, it is difficult to leave food behind, especially if it tastes good. So here is a tip: Take half the portion you usually take. When you've eaten that, stop and ask yourself "Am I still hungry?" If the answer is yes, take a second smaller portion, and then ask yourself the same question. When you are no longer hungry, stop eating. Wrap up the leftovers. They make a great lunch the following day, or dinner without cooking the next night, or even a snack if a few hours later you realize that you are hungry again.

The point is you have to retrain yourself to eat only until you are no longer hungry and fight nature to resist eating all the food in front of you. The fact is: The more food we eat the bigger our appetite and it doesn't even have to be food we really enjoy, simply what is within reach and hard to resist, which is why overeating is so dangerous. This is the reason you often eat that bagel at your meeting even when you do not feel hungry. But this is a behavior we can change and one of the ways to do that is to eliminate the visual cues we often respond to. For example, do not place serving containers on the table. Plate your meal at the counter and bring it to the table. Do this even with take-out. Or better yet, put the rest directly in the refrigerator since food left on the counter can also be a trigger. Another idea is to divide leftovers into meal-size portions, so you won't be tempted to "pick" and ruin a ready-made meal. You can even do this with a sandwich. Cut it in half, keep one half wrapped. Put the sandwich down between bites and after eating it, ask yourself if you are still hungry and really need to eat another quarter, but don't eat the whole sandwich just because it is there.

By the way, I'd like to think you have baby carrots as a side with that sandwich, but even if it is a bag of chips, eat the sandwich first to see if it satisfies you, if so, hold off on the chips. You can eat them at 4 p.m. when you get hungry again and possibly skip the candy bar you normally grab. Again, you are saving calories. In general, eating until you are no longer hungry, not full, is more comfortable. Besides saving calories, people report having more energy after meals. (Maybe walking the treadmill while watching your favorite show at 8 p.m. doesn't seem so daunting after all).

Cravings vs. Hunger

It is important to know the difference between cravings and hunger. A craving is wanting to eat in the absence of physical hunger. Eat only when you feel signs of hunger, a gnawing or growling stomach, lightheadedness, loss of focus, sometimes fatigue. Ask yourself "Am I hungry?" When the answer is no, it is a craving. Often, waiting just minutes to act on a craving will help it pass without acting on it. You can confront the craving with some self-talk and state the argument for not giving in. "I will not give in and get the ice cream because I want to ..." Or you can distract yourself from the craving by finding something else to do like taking a walk, tidying up, phoning a friend, meditating, or playing a game on your personal device.

One more alternative to soothe a craving is to introduce a new taste into your mouth. Most of us are reluctant to eat anything after we brush our teeth because the toothpaste alters the taste of anything we eat after brushing. Well, the next time you crave food without being hungry, brush your teeth! Breath spray also works if you can't brush.

A final thing to study from last week's food logs is the quality of your food choices. Meals and snacks need to be enjoyable, flavorful, and satisfying. And they also have to have variety and balance and be nutritious and calorie appropriate. A healthy body will lose weight easier than an unhealthy one. Assess your food choices. Look for particular foods you may be choosing that may have hidden calories. Cheese, sweets, salty snacks, fried foods, and convenience foods can add quite a lot of calories you may be unaware of. Don't despair. There are ways to cut down or make substitutions without eliminating them. It is not necessarily what we eat but how much that makes a difference. Look specifically for foods that added significant calories to the meal. Were these essential to your enjoyment of that meal? For instance, maybe that ham sandwich would have been just as satisfying with one slice of cheese instead of two, and you'd have saved 100 calories. Maybe skip the cheese on the turkey sandwich altogether. Maybe choose the turkey sandwich instead of the Italian hero and eliminate both the calories and the fat. Love pizza? Treat yourself once a week instead of twice. Snack on pretzels that are low in fat instead of high-fat chips and save 100–150 calories. Choose fruit for a sweet snack and skip the frosted donuts. Log all foods and beverages and watch your daily calorie totals go down. Do this and you'll see for yourself how easy it is to take in fewer calories by simply taking control over what and how much you eat by cutting back on high-calorie problem foods and controlling portion size.

Mind Your Peas and . . .

"Mindful Eating" is a term used to describe your state of mind when you are paying attention to what you are eating, when, where, how much, how it tastes, and whether or not it satisfies physically and emotionally. Writing down what you eat is your first step in changing from a mindless eater to a mindful eater. So, stop eating in front of the TV or at your desk, pay attention to what you are eating and eliminate distractions when you eat meals and snacks. Sitting down with a bag of chips instead of putting a portion in a bowl increases mindless eating. Changing these behaviors leads to feeling satisfied even when eating less.

The hunger/fullness scale helps you identify when you feel satisfied, but it only works when you give yourself a chance to pause and ask yourself if you should keep eating. To do this, make sure your plate only contains enough food for one serving at a time. This way you won't be tempted to eat more than you should while also providing yourself with time to stop and think after finishing the portion as to where you are on the hunger/fullness scale. Eating slowly is another effective mindful eating strategy. It doesn't matter if your meal is dashboard dining on take-out, or eating at the kitchen table, eating fast means consuming more calories per meal. Slowing down takes practice, but start by eating smaller bites, putting the fork down between bites, and chewing your food longer. Make this a new habit.

To practice mindful eating is to also be aware of how various foods affect your feelings, thoughts, and physical sensations. Take the time to tune into the temperature, texture, and taste of the food you are eating and the positive (or negative) thoughts and emotions generated by the experience.

This week your goal is to become a more mindful eater, so consciously start to consider where you eat, what is distracting you when you eat, and how your food is portioned. You also want to recognize what circumstances trigger you to overeat. Is it when you skip a meal or a snack? What are your high risk situations? Do you eat more at night? Do you eat when anxious or lonely? Do you eat as a reward? Are there foods you typically overeat? Take notice of what you are doing while eating and if it is distracting you from monitoring portion size, fullness level, satisfaction with the meal, or the taste and enjoyment of the food. Practicing mindfulness will help you identify the behaviors you need to change to decrease your calorie intake.

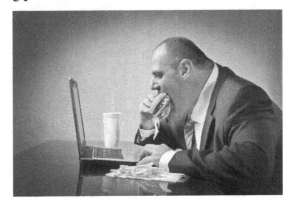

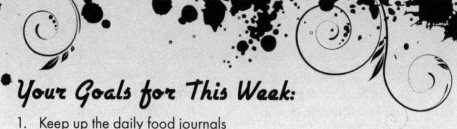

Your Goals for This Week:

1. Keep up the daily food journals

   a. Be mindful of when and in what circumstances you consume high-calorie foods or large portions

   b. Reduce, eliminate, or substitute high-calorie food choices you may not miss

2. Using the hunger/fullness scale, eat until you are satisfied not full

   a. Snack when meals are more than four hours apart or when your hunger level is near three on the scale

3. Keep up the daily activity journals

4. Wear an activity tracker or pedometer and aim to walk 10,000 steps every day

   a. Find ways to increase your ADLs

5. Increase your aerobic exercise

   a. Plan your walks, using the talk test to verify intensity

   b. Use aerobic exercise equipment, take fitness classes, go biking, or dance

   c. Make a list of activities and sports you enjoy now, those you enjoyed as a child, and those you seek to do when on vacation

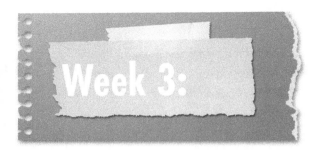

Calories Do Count

In my weight-loss classes, this is the point at which heads begin to nod when I ask about weight loss success and changes in behavior and attitude. But participants still insistent upon knowing, "How many calories a day am I supposed to be eating?" That is a valid question, but I first remind them to take a moment to acknowledge what they have accomplished so far.

Like those in my class, I'm hoping you can also count all of the following changes in your lifestyle and food behaviors as accomplishments.

- ▶ I record my food and beverage intake daily.

- ▶ I assess my intake and remove extra calories that I won't miss. I follow my internal hunger and fullness cues.

- ▶ I don't let myself get overly hungry and I don't eat more food than I am hungry for.

- ▶ I am more mindful when I eat, paying attention to the taste, amount, surroundings, and emotions to increase my satisfaction of the experience and to temper my portion control.

► I wear an activity tracker or pedometer and am finding more and more ways to increase my daily activity level. I am planning/implementing an exercise regimen suitable to my fitness level and lifestyle.

Behave!

I want to impress upon you that the changes you make in your behaviors throughout this ten-week plan are as essential to your weight loss and weight maintenance as your calorie counting, sometimes more. Behavior is what drives food choices, amounts, and outcomes. What we eat and how much we eat of it are often out of habit. We take our "usual" portion of a food, often without considering how hungry we are or how much of that food it will take to satisfy us. We just do it because that's how we always do it. We eat the entire candy bar or bowl of pasta without thinking or realizing that the taste became less enjoyable or that our hunger was gone.

Eating habits that support portion control and healthy choices, whether in your own kitchen, traveling, at a party, a ball game, or in a restaurant, will keep your calorie intake in check. Although it is not usually necessary to studiously calculate every calorie you consume during this program, I find that most people still question how many daily calories they should eat. The main reason that it is helpful to know is it adds to their understanding of how the calorie content of various foods relates to portion sizes regarding their "go to" food choices. Having this knowledge may also lead to establishing new habits pertaining to how often and how much you will eat of these favorite foods.

Establishing Good Habits

A habit is a behavior we do without thought and, unfortunately, this word is usually used in a negative way. In weight loss is has a particularly negative connotation when it is associated with undesirable behaviors, especially overeating. But now is the time to change how you feel about the word habit because you are now going to think of them as a way to change for the better. You are going to learn to replace those old unhealthy eating habits with healthy alternatives that will help you succeed in getting to your new healthy place as you learn to successfully integrate these new behaviors into your routine over time. This will be much easier than you think, and the good news is that it only takes between three weeks to three months to establish a new habit when you have a supportive physical and social environment. However, be aware that even the most well-meaning friends, spouses, or work environments can inadvertently sabotage your efforts by offering you tempting foods. There is no way around this, but if you are aware of potential pitfalls, it is easier to sidestep them, at least until your new habits are firmly established. Once a new habit becomes part of your daily life you can be proud because you've effectively instituted a real lifestyle change. It is with practice that a new behavior becomes a habit. It is by trial and correction that you choose a new behavior that will help you reach your goals, and it is practice that cements that behavior into a new habit. Of course, we are not infallible (that is why I did not say practice makes perfect). It is in the practicing that we stay focused. (Does a concert pianist or a baseball pitcher ever stop practicing?)

Journaling: Just Do It

If at this point you have been questioning whether you want to continue keeping a daily food log, then reconsider. Journaling is what will help you learn where, when, and which foods are providing how many calories. Journaling will help you figure out how much of those high-calorie foods you love to eat you can eat and still meet your calorie goal. The journal is going to point you toward how many calories you need to control your hunger, what time of day you may need more calories, what time of day you may need less. The journal will show you in what circumstances you tend to overdo it and help you preplan alternatives to avoid those sticky situations. So, clear your head, get rid of distractions, and grab a calculator. Got it? To make life easier, journal in the method you find easiest and most convenient. This way it will be easier to continually evaluate how your eating habits truly influence your weight and health.

How Many Calories?

It would be ideal if we all had access to an indirect calorimeter and a registered dietitian to assess our individual calorie needs, but some simple computations and honesty can provide you with a reasonable goal with which to work this plan. Why honesty? That's needed when assessing your activity level. But be forewarned: since a person who is moderately to very active burns more calories, a higher calorie intake will still support weight loss. However, if you overestimate your activity level—as most people tend to do—you will end up with a calorie goal that provides more calories than you burn and your weight loss efforts will be less effective.

"I was never aware of how many calories were in the portions and types of foods I was eating. By making a conscious effort to be aware of what I was consuming and regular exercise, I was able to lose over thirty pounds in almost twelve weeks. My blood pressure is normal again and my back and whole body are feeling much better. I still eat the foods that I like ... and many foods that I thought I would never enjoy and are actually healthy for you. I still enjoy going out to dinner and look and feel great! I even got my wife to lose a few pounds as she has been following my lead." Dennis

Calories are a measure of what we take in and what we burn off. Specifically, calories are a measure of the energy a food provides to the body as well as the energy the body uses. Our body is at work even when we are sleeping, or we wouldn't keep breathing, so we are constantly burning calories. But our activity level when awake increases our calorie needs and for our weight loss efforts, includes the calories we use from our daily intake as well as stored energy.

Here is a list of the calories per gram provided by the major components of foods:

Nutrient	Calories/gram of food
Carbohydrates	4
Proteins	4
Fats	9
Alcohol	7
Water, Vitamins/Minerals	0

If you eat the same number of calories you burn, then you maintain the same weight. If you eat more than you burn, then these additional calories are stored as body fat. But when you eat fewer calories than your body is using, creating a calorie deficit, it will draw from the stored calories to lose weight.

There are several methods to provide a rough estimate of total daily calorie needs to affect weight loss. You may choose one method or take an average of several results. Whatever your calorie goal is this week, an assessment at the end of the week will determine if your current one is appropriate or if a new goal has to be considered.

Determining Calorie Goals

Here are three ways to determine your calorie goals for losing one to two pounds per week, a healthy and realistic pace.

1. Calculate It the Way Dietitians Do

1. Divide your weight in pounds by 2.2 to convert it into kilograms.

2. Multiply your height in inches by 2.54 to convert it into centimeters.

3. Follow one of these gender-specific equations to determine your calorie needs at rest:

   Men: 10 x weight (kg) + 6.25 x height (cm) – 5 x age + 5

   Women: 10 x weight (kg) + 6.25 x height (cm) – 5 x age – 161[8]

4. To get the daily calorie range needed to maintain your current weight:

   If you're fairly sedentary, multiply the result from step #3 by 1.0 – 1.2.

   If you get 30 minutes of moderate-intensity aerobic activity most days or you reach 10,000 steps most days, multiply by 1.3 – 1.4.

   If you get 60 minutes of moderate- to high-intensity aerobic exercise most days, multiply by 1.4 – 1.6.

   This result is the range of calories that will maintain your current weight.

Use an online resource that does the calculations for you. Start by reducing calorie intake by twelve percent of your result. You will need to assess how appropriate your calorie intake is based on your activity and hunger level. [9]

2. Use a Quick-and-Rough Calculation Method

1. Divide your weight in pounds by 2.2 to convert it into kilograms.

2. Multiply this number by 25 to get the approximate calories you need daily to maintain your current weight. (Note: If you are more than 100 pounds over a healthy weight for your height or if you have a body mass index above 35, then multiply your weight in kilograms by 20 instead of 25.)

3. Or calculate your calorie needs by checking out an online calorie calculator that uses the Harris-Benedict Method.

4. Reduce the resulting calorie level by twelve percent as your starting calorie goal and continue to assess activity and hunger levels and adjust when necessary.

"The light turned on for me was when I calculated how many calories I needed to stick to in order to lose weight. I also liked learning how to read food labels, restaurant nutrition downloads, and meal planning because they made me realize how badly I had been feeding myself and my family."

Norman

3. Estimate Calories Based on Statistics

Most often, women lose weight by limiting themselves to 1,200–1,500 calories per day, while men can take in 1,600–1,900. A moderately-to-very-active person should aim for the upper end of those ranges. (Moderately active is defined as someone who sustains aerobic exercise for thirty to sixty minutes on five or more days each week.)

Whichever method you use, you must settle on a realistic goal. If you're a man who found that you usually eat 2,600 calories a day and are just beginning a walking program, cutting that to 1,600 calories may be unrealistic and unnecessary. You might consider reducing calorie intake to 2,300, and when comfortable with that drop it to 1,900 calories, while increasing your activity level at the same time. On the other hand, a woman who has been restricting her calories to 1,400 for years may want to consider maintaining a 1,400 daily calorie goal but concentrate most of her efforts on increasing her exercise.

You may want to assess your calorie needs using two of or all three methods, then use an average or choose the one that you feel most comfortable with.

Here's an example: Jane is 200 pounds. According to her pedometer she walks about 5,000 steps each day in her routine activities of daily life. In addition, she has finished her first five nights of walking for thirty minutes after dinner.

▶ *Using the calculation method, Jane requires 2,272 calories a day and therefore needs a goal of 2000 calories to lose one to two pounds per week.*

▶ *Using the estimation method, Jane would choose 1,500 calories a day as a limit.*

I would suggest that Jane should average the two methods and choose a goal of 1750 calories per day as her limit.

Also keep in mind that as you lose weight, you need to continually reassess calorie goals because when you weigh less, you may also need to lower calorie intake to continue losing weight. A significant weight loss also reduces the need for energy, which in turn translates to needing fewer daily calories. Researchers have discovered that a 20-pound loss from a calorie restricted diet requires eating an average of 100 calories less per day. Don't be fooled by this seemingly small number of extra calories because they can slowly add up to a weight gain of five- to ten-pounds over the course of *one* year. Once again, let hunger be your guide and recalculate your portion habits accordingly. However, if you have not been basing your portion sizes on your internal hunger/satiety cues, I recommend you start using any of the three methods listed above.

Also consider that it may not be your calorie intake that's the issue but the time of day you get most of your calories, the ratio of carbs, fats, and proteins you eat (stay tuned for more on that), or that you are not consistent with your caloric intake. For example, getting 1,400 calories one day, 1,900 the next, then 1,200 calories. This yo-yo eating promotes calorie storage as body fat.

It is imperative that you never set a calorie goal below 1,200 calories unless a physician recommends it and provides monitored care. This rule supersedes any calculations. Why? Below 1,200 calories a day, your metabolism slows, and you run the risk of losing lean body mass. Neither consequence is healthy, and both impede weight loss.

Assess your food and activity journals each week to help determine if you have chosen the daily calorie goal that's right for you. Were you excessively hungry between meals at that calorie level? Are you mildly to moderately hungry four hours after meals? Are your snacks appropriate? Are you reaching your activity goals? Are you losing one to two pounds per week? These questions won't be easily answered after only one week. Remember, habits take at least three weeks to establish. After two weeks, though, if you have not lost one to two pounds, reassess your calorie intake and calories burned at your current activity level.

Time of day is also a factor in how energy is burned or stored. A common problem is eating a lot of your calories late in the day. Why is it a good idea to break this habit? Taking in more than a third of your daily calories when you tend to be less active promotes fat storage.

The Art of Balancing

As you calculate your calorie intake food by food and meal by meal, you'll notice which starchy foods you are eating in abundance and how many calories are from high-fat foods (even healthful ones, like nuts) and foods that are high in added fats, like a buttered roll. That's not to say that these foods should be avoided. Nuts, for example, have been shown to aid weight loss, but only if you stick to a small portion a day, typically one-quarter cup. Once you learn to control the amounts of high-calorie foods and balance them with the lower-calorie foods you eat, it will be easier to meet your calorie goals for weight loss.

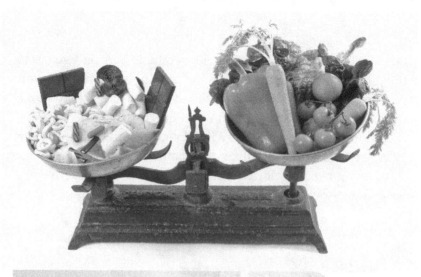

The Importance of Fiber

A diet high in fiber-rich foods—vegetables, fruits, and whole grains—is scientifically proven to control weight, improve blood pressure, lower cholesterol, and reduce the risk of developing a myriad of medical conditions. Foods that are high in fiber from plant-based sources and these foods are referred to as complex carbohydrates, whereas plant-based foods that have been processed and stripped of fiber, like white flour, sugar, and fruit juices, are called simple carbohydrates. Eating high-fiber foods also has the added bonus of helping you to feel fuller even when lowering calorie intake.

Remember that there really are no forbidden foods when you know how to balance a high-calorie lunch with a low-calorie dinner. In the mood for a burger tonight? Fine. Then have grilled chicken over a salad for lunch with low-fat dressing. And don't forget to add some fiber in the form of beans, lentils, or peas to the salad. Don't forget that you also need to include at least one carbohydrate serving with each meal to ensure satisfaction and fuel for the body. This means that sometimes you might want to skip the bread and save an extra serving of carbohydrates to treat yourself to a few French fries. Balancing helps you do that.

Carbs, Fat, and Protein: Does It Really Matter?

Yes, the percentage of calories you take in from carbohydrates, proteins, and fats is as critical as your daily calorie intake. Research shows that a moderate carbohydrate restriction is beneficial for weight loss.[10] Severe carbohydrate restrictions, however, may have adverse health effects. Most registered dietitians recommend that 45 percent to 50 percent of food intake be from carbohydrates, mostly as whole grains or legumes. To determine how much is right for you, take 50 percent of your daily calorie goal and divide by 4 to get the maximum grams of carbohydrates you need per day.

For example: Jane's goal is 1,400 calories per day with up to 700 calories from carbohydrates; therefore, Jane's daily need of carbohydrates is not more than 175 grams per day.

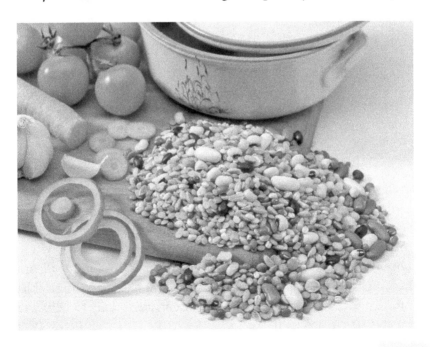

For foods that are commonly eaten in large quantities, web-based food journals like the myfitnesspal app can also keep track of your daily carbohydrate totals as well as your carbohydrate intake for each meal.

If you are not using a web-based format for journaling, choose the sample journal on the next page to create your own daily food and activity log or download a PDF of the food and activity log at www.LoseItfortheLastTime.com to record the fruit, vegetable, milk/yogurt, and starch servings you consume daily to make it easier to meet your daily-serving goals.

Foods That Contain Carbohydrates

Foods are characterized by which nutrient they have the most of. Therefore, fruit, vegetables, milk, yogurt, corn, peas, beans, lentils, rice, pasta, bread, cereal, and potatoes are carbs. Here's a general daily guide for a healthy diet:

- ► *2–4 servings of* **fruit**

- ► *5–8 servings of* **vegetables**

- ► *2–3 servings of* **low-fat milk or yogurt**

- ► *6–11 servings* **whole grains, beans, legumes (peas, lentils), and starchy vegetables**

Take a look at the daily food log on the next page. (Use the sample log on the next page to create your own daily food and activity log for weeks three through ten or download a PDF of the food and activity log for weeks three through ten at www.LoseItfortheLastTime.com.) You will be using this food log from now on. There are places to record the number of fruit, vegetable, milk/yogurt, and starch servings you consume daily to help you meet your chosen goal.

Name_____ DAILY JOURNAL Date_____

My eating goals _____

My exercise goals _____

Time	Food eaten	Amount	Calories	Servings Eaten					
				Starch	Milk/Yogurt	Fruit	Vegetables	Protein	Fat
	TOTAL CALORIES:								

ACTIVITY LOG

Time	Activity	Minutes	Steps

One Serving of Starch Equals

▶ *1/2 cup of potatoes, cereal, or starchy vegetables*

▶ *1/3 cup rice or pasta*

▶ *One slice of bread*

▶ *1/2 cup beans or lentils*

If you were to choose to eat one cup of rice for dinner, you'd be eating three starches. If you ate a half cup of cold cereal with eight ounces nonfat milk and a small banana (one starch, one milk/yogurt, one fruit) or two slices of toast and eight ounces of low-fat yogurt (two starches, one milk/yogurt), in each breakfast you would be consuming three servings of carbohydrates. Use the food journal to monitor your carbohydrate intake. A mild carbohydrate restriction will assist you in weight loss. Keeping track of your carbs also will help you control your portion sizes and tell you where you tend to overeat starchy foods. By the way, the pasta in your weekly pasta dinner is not what's keeping you from losing weight; it is how much pasta you are likely piling on your plate. Remember, it is often not what you eat but how much you eat that makes the difference.

For many people, carbs are the most difficult to portion control. And keep in mind that lots of carbs are hidden. Take a look at ingredient lists and nutrition labels. Every fifteen grams of carbohydrates you see listed is the equivalent of a serving of bread. Chances are you have not been counting all those carbohydrate servings, so start now by checking your salad dressing, sauces, and even packaged fish and chicken as they can also contain hidden starches and sugars.

For now, determine your daily intake of fruit, milk/yogurt, vegetables, and starches, especially whole grains, that meet 50 percent of your daily calorie goal.[11] Take the week to learn where your carbohydrate sources are and what time of day is most satisfying to include them. It could be that you're more satisfied eating more starches at breakfast and dinner. You may find you need to munch your way through your late afternoon and popcorn serves you better than a sandwich roll at lunch. Use trial and correction until a meal pattern emerges that suits you best. There is time to navigate your way through fats and proteins later. Remember, when it comes to food, one size does not fit all. You are finding your own path, your weight goal, the destination.

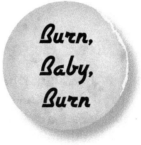

Burn, Baby, Burn

— or —

Making Fitness as Important as Going to the Doctor or the Hair Salon

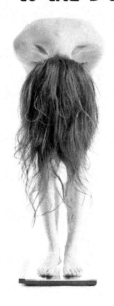

What about the other side of the weight loss equation? You now have a clearer plan for reducing calorie intake. But keep in mind that greater physical activity will burn more calories, so you'll lose faster. To do so, you'll need to constantly refine your exercise plan. The walking program you started is a lifestyle approach. Recording your steps each day shows small changes in activity level and every bit helps. But try to do more all the time. Count things you may not consider exercise. Walking to do your errands or going to the mall requires extra steps. For example: The day turned cool yesterday and I was encouraged to stack firewood, certainly not an everyday activity, but extra exercise I can add to the forty minutes of aerobics I had accomplished that morning. And on top of burning calories and increasing metabolism, exercise improves blood pressure, cholesterol, and blood sugar. It improves mood, self-esteem, and confidence. Exercise is also important during weight loss because it preserves muscle mass, sometimes lost along with fat during weight loss.

Exercising to Burn Calories

Exercise has three parameters, duration, frequency, and intensity. Increasing any one, or a combination of two or all three, will increase the number of calories you burn, the muscle you build, and improve your health and fitness levels. The following are ways to ease yourself into getting more from the exercise routines you are already doing!

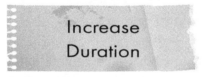

Increase
Duration

If you are walking, biking, or playing basketball for fifteen-minute-a-day, increase the time a mere five minutes to twenty minutes.

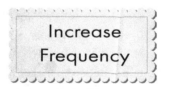

Increase
Frequency

If you are walking thirty minutes for three days every week, increase the frequency of your walks to four days a week.

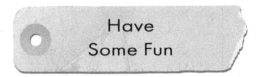

Increase Intensity

If you are walking at a pace that covers a mile in thirty minutes, up your pace to cover that mile in twenty-five minutes, then twenty.

Have Some Fun

This coming week try adding one or more physical recreational activities. Start by taking a look at the list you made last week of activities you thought you'd enjoy for ideas. For example, perhaps you wanted to take a bike ride with your kid. How about scheduling that nature walk you've been putting off. What about signing up for that martial arts or dance class you've been interested in trying. Think about making good on your friend's invitation to play tennis.

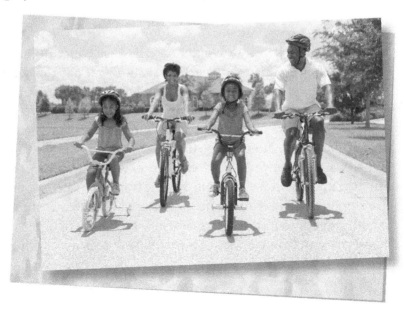

Make an Appointment with Yourself to Exercise

Instead of using your busy life as an excuse not to be active schedule a time with yourself to exercise. It works! At the beginning of each week you need to set these appointments to exercise in your calendar. Just as you record your doctor or hair salon appointments, you must treat your exercise time with the same respect—and not cancel or ignore it. Consider how much more you can accomplish if you are stronger, lighter, and less fatigued. Taking the time to exercise actually improves your productivity, your mood, and your energy.

Improve Incrementally

If you don't feel physically ready for long exercise sessions or if your lifestyle or job truly presents barriers to having the time to exercise, then try integrating activities into your day that also count as exercise. For instance, instead of trying to find the time for a forty minute walk, try working short walks, say twenty minutes long, before lunch and maybe another walk for twenty minutes after work. No time for the gym, so check out YouTube for that fitness class you really want to take. This way you can do it at home any time. Peleton, NordicTrac, and Mirror offer subscription services to home fitness classes and other streaming content. In addition, there are many home exercise options for all skill levels and budgets for a wide variety of activities, with or without equipment.

Set Realistic Goals

To make the above suggestions a reality, you need to develop a realistic exercise plan that works for you. Your goals also have to be realistic, measurable, and obtainable. What we're after here are short-term efforts because they in turn lead to short-term success, which ultimately lead to long-term goal achievement. Choose your goals for the coming week that are doable and will increase your physical activity. Just because you can walk a mile in twenty or thirty minutes does not mean you need to exercise like you are training for the next marathon, instead walk six days a week or choose to walk forty minutes a day as your goal. With each incremental improvement you are closer to your long-term goal. And remember, that when you maintain a new behavior over time it establishes new, healthy habits.

By influencing your energy balance through the combination of eating less and moving more, you will enjoy bigger results. For motivation consider that: People who exercise have the greatest long-term success at weight loss. So get moving!

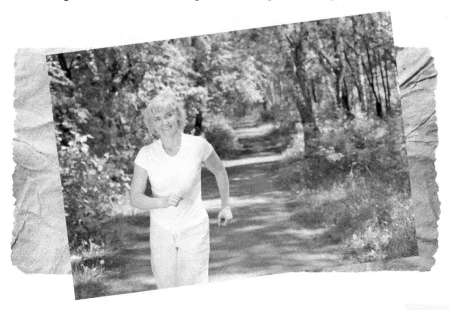

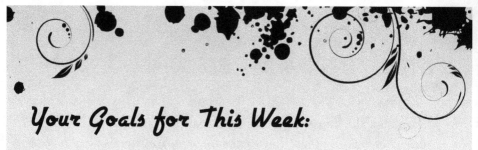

Your Goals for This Week:

1. Record what you eat in your food journal every day, including:

   a. *Noting your calorie goal and striving to eat that same amount each day*

   b. *Noting your carbohydrate goal and attempt to meet that goal each day*

   c. *Keeping an eye on the number of carbohydrate servings and striving to meet the recommendations for a balanced diet*

   d. *Eat at least 1–2 fruits and 3–5 vegetable servings each day*

2. Keep a record of your physical activity:

   a. *Pay attention to your activity tracker or pedometer goal every day*

   b. *Meet or exceed your steps/day from the previous day (Plan your exercise goal for the week.)*

   c. *Meet or exceed your planned exercise goal*

   d. *Consider altering the frequency, duration, and intensity of your exercise sessions*

3. Continue to practice mindful eating behaviors:

    a. *Take less on your plate*

    b. *Follow hunger/fullness cues*

    c. *Balance high-calorie food choices with lower calorie foods*

(If you are not using a web-based format, you can create your own food and activity log for using the samples on page 53 as a guide or download a PDF of the food and activity log at www.LoseItfortheLastTime.com.)

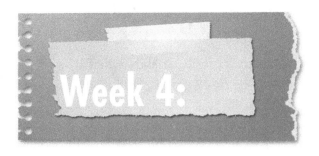

Week 4:

Weighing In on Carbs, Proteins, and Fats

It is now time for you to do an honest self-assessment of your realistic, doable, measurable, achievable goals. During these past three weeks, you have traveled quite a distance on your path to wellness by using the tools you have been given to change your eating and physical activity habits. It's now time to take stock of your progress and ask yourself:

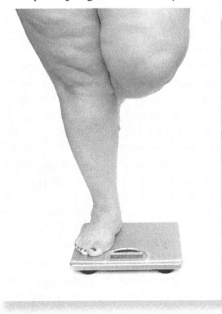

- ▶ *Am I measuring my progress by keeping accurate food and activity journals?*

- ▶ *Have I made the adjustments in calorie intake, time of day I eat, and the amount and type of carbohydrate I consume?*

- ▶ *Am I losing one to two pounds each week?*

If you aren't losing weight, my experience shows that it is probably because you are doing one or more of the following:

- *Not walking or exercising consistently*

- *Fluctuating intake of several hundred calories from one day to the next*

- *Skipping meals or snacks*

- *Consuming the majority of calories after 5:00 p.m.*

- *Eating a high intake of high-sugar, high-fat sweet snacks*

- *Dining out a lot or getting take-out, both of which makes it difficult to correctly count calories (I saw one woman mistakenly log 1 cup of fried rice as 250 calories when it should have been 1000 calories)*

- *Not eating enough calories throughout the day to keep your body from creating a starvation state*

Consistent Behavior = Continued Weight loss

If you are not losing weight, look through your journals and try to identify what you need to adjust, work on, or modify. Remember too, that it is always okay to stop where you are to catch your breath and make any necessary adjustments before moving on. The important thing to always keep in mind is that it's the short-term efforts that lead to long-term success. So turn your efforts into habits that become permanent changes in behavior because these changes are vital to continued weight loss and weight maintenance.

If, however, after carefully practicing these new behaviors you find you are not losing appreciable weight, HAVE NO FEAR. You may be one of the frustrated few. Some bodies need time to adjust to changes. Keep in mind that you may have been abusing your body's regulatory systems for quite some time and your brain hasn't had time to readjust and is fighting to keep things constant. Don't let this get you down. STICK TO YOUR PLAN. If you are consistent in your calorie intake and diligent in your goals to increase the duration, frequency, and intensity of your daily walking or exercise plan, YOU WILL LOSE WEIGHT.

At the beginning of her weight-loss program, a woman participant was skeptical about the outcome. Her way of participating meant sitting with her arms folded across her chest and questioning the success of many of the techniques being discussed. In spite of saying she was disappointed in losing just three pounds, it was still enough for her to enjoy the way her clothes now fit and that her blood sugars were better controlled. Just experiencing these small benefits was enough of an incentive for her to commit to continuing these new behaviors. Her choice to continue was rewarded further because she began to lose even more weight without making any additional changes. When I last spoke to her, she shared with me her joy at having lost twenty pounds after completing the program. Learning healthy habits and sticking with them works.

Planning the Plate: Portion Control the Easy Way

I would now like to introduce a technique to make it easier to implement portion control. Earlier I introduced the nutrient carbohydrates, and even devised a method of breaking down these nutrients into food groups, non-starchy vegetables, fruit, starches, and so on, but now I want to show you a concept called Planning the Plate that is designed to help you plan your meal so that you eat from all the food groups in the correct proportion, a great tool for creating well-balanced meals. This technique works because:

▶ *Planning the Plate helps you learn about various food groups and their recommended portion size at each meal in relation to the other foods included in that meal. Take a look at the planning-the-plate diagram for breakfast and the one for lunch and dinner. Portion sizes are indicated by what proportion of the plate the food group occupies.*

▶ *Planning the Plate allows you to eat the foods you want and still include the nutrient-rich food your body needs.*

▶ *Planning the Plate makes it possible to eat more and still lose weight because your plate is loaded with only high-quality calories.*

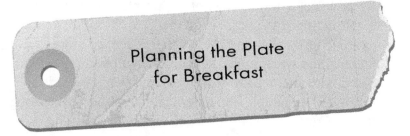

Planning the Plate
for Breakfast

Begin by taking a look at the plate diagram, notice that one quarter is devoted to complex carbohydrates in the form of starches like high-fiber cereal, whole grain bread potatoes, brown rice, and beans. The second quarter of the plate holds a serving of fruit. The third quarter contains lean protein and protein sourced from milk and yogurt. The final quarter is for vegetables and a small serving of fat.

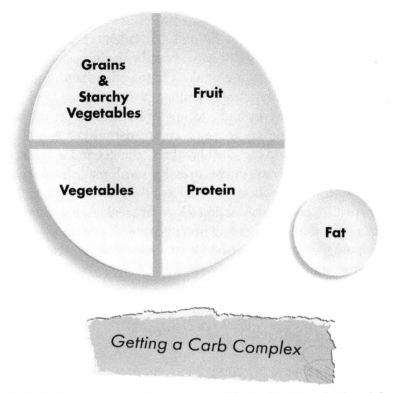

Getting a Carb Complex

Carbohydrates are our best source of fuel which is why breakfast foods tend to be carbohydrates.

Eating carbohydrates for breakfast supplies the body with the fuel it needs after a period of sleep and not eating. In fact, carbohydrates are the only food source of energy the brain can utilize. Just as you can't expect your car to run without fuel, you can't expect your body and brain to function without the carb-essential part of a healthy breakfast.

Good Carbs/Bad Carbs

The main sources of carbohydrates commonly eaten at breakfast can be simple or complex.

Eating simple carbohydrates, like sugar, causes a high insulin response which makes the body tired and hungry as opposed to energizing it. This is why eating sugar-laden breakfast cereals or pastries are not a good way to start the day, especially if you are trying to control calorie intake. On the other hand, complex carbohydrates like whole grains contain fiber and provide a long-lasting source of energy and a feeling of fullness, so are the better choice. Now you know why a cup of oatmeal or two slices of whole grain bread are ideal breakfast choices and a donut or muffin is not. So, always say yes to eating meals made from whole grains with fiber because not only are they lower in sugar, but they are also lower in fat. Eating a low-fat breakfast also saves on calories not to mention being heart healthy. If you find yourself feeling sluggish after eating breakfast, chances are you can blame it on your choice of menu.

Protein Power

Protein is another important component of a healthy breakfast.

▶ *Protein makes you feel more satisfied after eating.*

▶ *Protein replaces carb and fat calories and aids in weight loss;*

▶ *Protein eaten at every meal makes it easier to meet your total protein goal for the day.*

Eating protein for breakfast can be tricky if you're not sure which foods are the best sources. When you think of protein, it's usually chicken, fish, beef, pork, beans, and maybe tofu that come to mind, but these foods aren't appetizing breakfast food choices for everyone. However, there are many more protein-rich choices from which to choose to start your day that may be more appealing to you. For example, low-fat cheese, eggs or egg substitutes, peanut butter, lox, or other fish. Also, do not forget that eight ounces of low-fat milk or six ounces of low-fat yogurt contain 8 grams of protein. Greek yogurts contain about 15 grams of protein which counts as the entire protein portion of the plate. (Note that foods that contain more than one nutrient count as more than one place on the plate. For example, milk counts as both starch and protein and eggs as both protein and fat.)

Protein powders, though not considered a whole unprocessed food, may be beneficial when whole foods are not an option. In this case, a better option is to choose pure pea or whey protein powder instead of a flavored protein powder mix with added sugar. A great tasting and balanced high-protein morning meal would be a fruit smoothie made with yogurt, milk or milk substitute, fruit, and protein powder. Also check out protein enhanced breakfast mixes, such as the high protein oatmeal made by Quaker and the high protein pancake and waffle mixes produced by Kodiak Cakes and Birch Bender. Because protein is also often thought of as a main component of lunch and dinner meals, you'll learn more about protein later in this chapter.

Fat Chance

When you look closely at the plate diagram you'll see that there is only a fraction of space allowed for fat. This is because fat is high in calories and eating too much of it promotes heart disease, so it's best consumed in small portions. Healthy fats, such as nuts added to oatmeal or yogurt, or a sliced avocado served

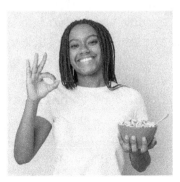

over eggs or on toast, are all tasty choices. When choosing breakfast options consider that your wisest choices are the morning meals you enjoy eating that also have the added benefit of being low in fat allowing you to save your fat calories for lunch and dinner when you may enjoy them the most.

Breakfast Menus Sampler

1-2 eggs (or 3 egg whites), 1/2 cup spinach, 1-2 slices whole grain bread,1 cup strawberries, 6 ounces low-fat or fat-free yogurt

1 cup cooked oatmeal, 8 ounces nonfat milk, 2 tbs. raisins

1 whole grain English muffin, 1 tbsp. peanut butter, 1/2 sliced banana, 1 low-fat string cheese, 6-ounce low-sodium V-8 juice

1 4-inch tortilla, 1/2 cup beans, 1 ounce 2 percent milk cheddar cheese, 1/4 cup chopped tomatoes or jarred salsa, 1 cup melon

If your meal plan allows for more than 300–350 calories at breakfast, you may increase your portion sizes, but stay with the same food groups and keep them in the same proportions. It's not

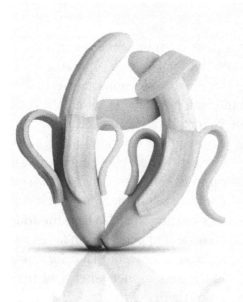

uncommon for a person with greater calorie needs to increase the starch and/or protein portion by one or two servings and that is exactly what I do not want you to do. Proportions are important.

But what do you do if you are trying to stick to 1,200 calories a day or not hungry enough to eat a full plate at breakfast? How do you then plan to include food from all food groups to insure you are eating a balanced nutritious diet? The answer is to eat a mid-morning snack. Snacking gives you the perfect opportunity to eat from the food group you missed at breakfast. For example, you could grab a low-fat or fat-free yogurt, a piece of fruit, and/or one cup raw vegetables to make up for an abbreviated breakfast.

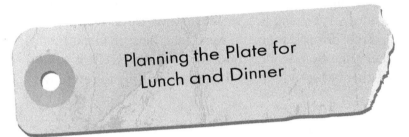

Planning the Plate for Lunch and Dinner

Lunch and dinner plates differ from the breakfast plate because the body has different nutrition requirements as the day progresses. For these two meals, notice that vegetables make up half the meal. Cooked or raw, vegetables are the food highest in nutrients and the lowest in calories. Eating one-half cup of a cooked non-starchy vegetable, such as green beans, broccoli, or spinach

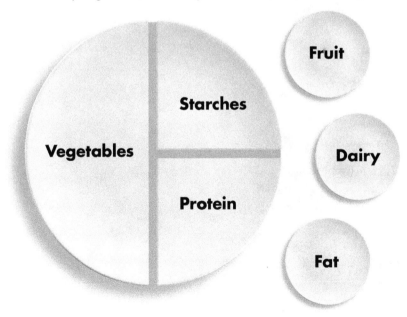

or one cup of raw carrots, cucumbers, tomatoes, or greens equals only twenty-five calories. (See below for a non-starchy vegetable list.) This leaves the remainder of the plate divided equally between starch and protein with a small amount of space devoted to fat.

Fruit and milk/yogurt are often served separately, but feel free to add your fruit serving to a salad, stew, or sauce. However, if you skip fruit or milk/yogurt at mealtime, be sure to eat them at another time. Remember, these foods make excellent snack choices either between lunch and dinner or during the evening.

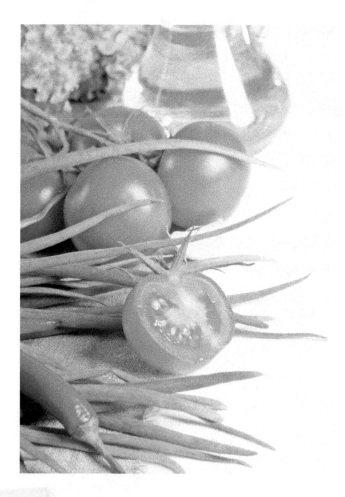

NON-STARCHY VEGETABLES

Artichokes

Arugula

Asparagus

Beets

Broccoli

Broccoli rabe

Brussels sprouts

Cabbage

Carrots

Cauliflower

Celery

Cucumber

Eggplant

Endive

Fennel (Anise)

Green beans

Greens (Kale, Swiss chard, Mustard)

Leeks

Lettuce

Mushrooms

Okra

Onion

Peppers

Radish

Sauerkraut

Scallions (green onions)

Shallots

Snow peas (pea pods)

Spinach

Summer (yellow) squash

Tomato (fresh and canned)

Tomatillos

Turnips

Water chestnuts

Watercress

Wax beans

Zucchini

A Full Plate with Fewer Calories

We tend to eat the same volume of food from day to day no matter how dense the calories. The key then to controlling hunger while losing or maintaining weight loss is to be satisfied without increasing the amount you eat. This means you have no choice but to replace high-calorie foods with lower-calorie choices when trying to lose weight. Eating more vegetables at meals adds volume so the overall calorie intake is lower. This added volume also guarantees you will be satisfied after a meal. Going hungry or feeling deprived is counterproductive to any weight loss effort as you no doubt already know. If you find this happening to you then choose foods containing high water content because water content lowers calorie density and increases portion size for the same number of calories. For example, a cup of broth-based soup is more satisfying than eating four to five crackers and eating fifteen grapes is more satisfying than eating eight almonds.

In fact, this idea of eating high-volume foods for satiety has been researched by Barbara Rolls, PhD at Penn State University, and is discussed at length in her book *Volumetrics*.[12] Dr. Rolls

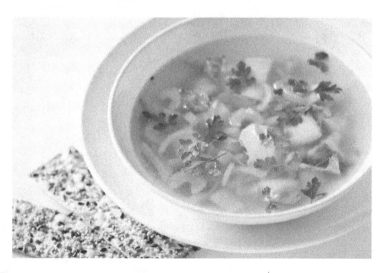

made this discovery in the laboratory when she noticed that participants who ate food with a high water volume and low-calorie density were more satisfied. This means that you can reduce calorie intake without going hungry while enjoying larger portions. To practice this way of eating, all you need to do is increase your intake of vegetables, fruits, low-fat milk/yogurt, soups and stews, beans and legumes, and decrease your portion sizes for cheese, nuts, high-fat protein, butter, oil, chips, crackers, and cookies. Do this and you will be eating a satisfying and larger volume of food while losing weight. Yes, you read this correctly, filling your meals with low-calorie dense foods means you can eat more than you are eating today and still lose weight.

The easiest and best way to determine calorie density of any food is by reading the package label. Choose those foods whose calories are less than the grams per serving. (For example, 6-inch banana, 101g, contains 90 calories). However, use caution when choosing foods whose calories are equal to or up to twice the number of grams. (3 ounces salmon, 84g, has 84 calories). When the calories are more than twice the number of grams, limit your intake. (1 cup, 41g, cold cereal has 170 calories).

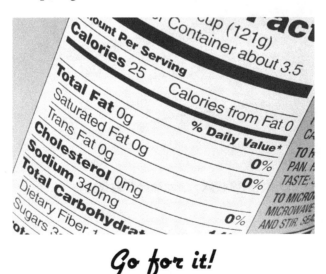

Go for it!

Nutrition Facts

Serving Size 1/4 Cup (30g)
Servings Per Container About 38

Amount Per Serving

Calories 200 Calories from Fat 150

	% Daily Value*
Total Fat 17g	
Saturated Fat 2.5g	26%
Trans Fat 0g	13%
Cholesterol 0mg	
Sodium 120mg	0%
Total Carbohydrate 7g	5%
Dietary Fiber 2g	2%
Sugars 1g	8%
Protein 5g	

Vitamin A 0%	•	Vitamin C 0%
Calcium 4%	•	Iron 8%

*Percent Daily Values are based on a 2,000 calorie diet.

Just Say Whoa!

Foods with Low Calorie Density

- Low-fat yogurt

- Fat-free cottage cheese

- Instant oatmeal prepared with water

- Beans

- Peas

- Lentils

- Tofu

- Corn

- Bananas

- Sweet potatoes

- White Potatoes

- Fish

- Grapes

- Olives

- Avocados

- Fat-free salad dressing

- Fat-free sour cream

- Fat-free mayonnaise

- Ketchup

- High-fiber, low-sugar cereal with nonfat milk

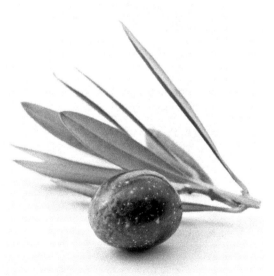

Foods with Very Low Calorie Density

- Carrots
- Cucumbers
- Celery
- Chicken broth
- Lettuce
- Tomatoes
- Asparagus
- Broccoli
- Grapefruit
- Strawberries
- Fat-free vinaigrette
- Vegetable soup
- Watermelon
- Cantaloupe

- Winter squash
- Peaches
- Apples
- Blueberries
- Oranges
- Mushrooms
- Peppers
- Raspberries
- Pears
- Zucchini
- Spinach

Liquid Calories

Several studies have shown that eating a broth-type soup or low-fat salad prior to a meal reduces calorie intake for the whole meal. This means that when trying to reduce the calorie density of a meal the water content must be gotten from the food itself and not drunk separately from a glass or bottle. Likewise, and contrary to popular belief, drinking water before or during a meal, although healthy, will not reduce hunger. Drinking beverages is also not helpful when trying to lose weight as hunger and thirst are regulated by separate mechanisms. This is why you need to take into account the number of calories in sugary beverages like juice, soda, or presweetened iced tea because if you don't make an adjustment in your daily food intake to account for those extra calories you will gain weight.

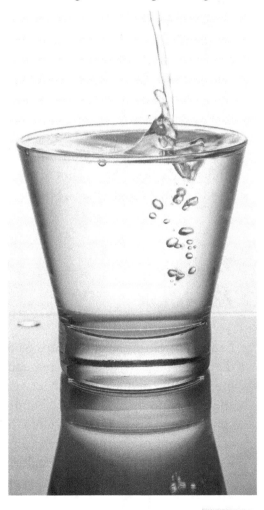

Now is a good time to talk frankly about how added calories from beverage choices hinder weight loss efforts. We all know that sugar-packed regular soda (9 teaspoons for every 12 ounces) is not good for your waistline, teeth, or bones. Now brace yourself because this also applies to coffee. Most people are not aware that one 16-ounce light and sweet coffee adds 133 calories to their morning meal. For heavy coffee drinkers, that's almost 400 calories a day. Over the course of a year this adds up to a significant number of (empty) calories that can pack on more than just a few pounds. You would have to walk between four and five miles every day just to burn them off. Sports drinks, like Gatorade, may be important if you engage in 60 minutes or more of sustained physical activity and need to replenish with the electrolytes and carbohydrates found in these drinks, but most of us need only water to rehydrate. The calories in alcohol, too, also trip up many people. Consider that one can of beer contains 150 calories with a six-pack netting 900 calories. One shot of vodka or gin is 100 calories, and that's without the added the calories from the juice, soda, or cocktail mixes. Portion sizes, too, also come into play here and are often the culprit. Sodas once came in 6 ½-ounce bottles, today a 20-ounce bottle is the norm. A typical glass of wine is often 6-ounces, up from 4 ounces. And the average bartender adds more than a shot of liquor when mixing a martini or mojitos. The bottom line is: Stick to calorie-free beverages.

Proteins Revisited

Eating protein-rich foods keeps us feeling fuller longer because they take longer to digest, increase the production of satiety hormones (the chemical messengers that signal when you've had enough), and reduce levels of hunger hormones, all of which contribute to lowering total calorie intake. It also takes a significant amount of energy to chew, digest, and metabolize protein which translates into burning calories. The energy cost in consuming and processing proteins is up to three times higher than eating the equivalent number of calories from carbs or fats. What is important for you to know is that protein contains the same four calories per gram as carbohydrates, but fewer calories are stored from protein.

This doesn't mean that you can eat proteins without discretion and not put on weight. Consuming too many calories from any food source adds to your body's fat stores. But eating too much protein has other consequences as it overworks the kidneys that rid the body of excess nitrogen byproducts and weakens the bones by depleting the body of calcium. Yet, it is important to eat an adequate amount of protein because the body needs it for cell growth and repair, hormone production, and a strong immune system. Eating protein also aids in muscle recovery, but that may have more to do with when the protein is eaten rather than with the amount.

High protein intake also aids weight loss by increasing metabolism and preserving lean body mass (muscle), in addition to adding to the feeling of satiety when cutting back on fat and carbs.

How Much is Enough

The US Dietary Reference Intakes sets the **minimum** protein requirement at 15% (67.5 grams for an 1,800-calorie diet) and an upper limit at 35% of total calorie intake (157 grams for an 1,800-calorie diet). Although most adults consume more than the minimum recommended, protein needs do vary depending on gender, activity level, and body composition. For example, body builders, those who perform endurance sports, and pregnant women need more.

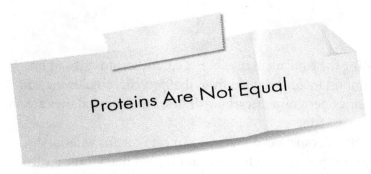

Proteins Are Not Equal

Because protein can come from a variety of sources, it goes without saying that their calorie counts also vary. Below is an overview to help you in choosing lean proteins that are good not only for your waist, but also for your heart health:

- **Animal proteins** Beef, pork, and cheese are high in fat and, therefore, have more calories per ounce than skinless chicken breasts and fish. Even a whole egg, with its seventy-five calories, is much higher than eating the equivalent amount of protein that can be gotten from eating two egg whites that contain a total of thirty-five calories.

- **Plant proteins** Beans, legumes (including peanuts), and soy provide adequate healthy protein while adding disease-fighting nutrients but the protein from vegetables and tree nuts is much lower (only one to two grams) and would have to be consumed in very large quantities to be an appreciable source.

- **Dairy** These products are a sensible protein source, especially when you choose the low- or fat-free varieties of milk, yogurt, and cheese. The key is to get the protein without the fat because one ounce of regular cheese is usually eighty to one hundred calories compared to an ounce of reduced-fat cheese (made from 2-percent milk or marked part-skim) with forty-five to fifty calories.

Calculating Your Protein Needs

Go back to the planning-the-plate diagram and see what fraction protein takes up on the plate relative to vegetables and starches. Consider that one serving is one ounce of animal protein, one egg, a half cup beans/legumes or eight ounces of milk/yogurt. Your daily protein intake will be based on your daily calorie goal.

For an average-size adult, the amount of protein in a healthy daily meal plan usually includes:

1–2 servings of protein at breakfast

> *(example: 3 egg whites)*

1 serving protein with a fruit or starch mid-morning

> *(example: 1-ounce low-fat cheese with a small apple)*

3–6 servings of protein at lunch

> *(example: 4 ounces grilled chicken)*

1 serving of protein with a fruit or starch mid-afternoon

> *(example: 1 ounce tuna with whole grain crackers)*

4–6 servings of protein at dinner

> *(example: 4 ounces salmon)*

For women, especially those on a 1,200–1,300 daily calorie plan, the protein need is at the lower end of the range. For example, one serving of low-fat or fat-free milk or yogurt at either breakfast or mid-morning, and three to four ounces of lean animal protein at lunch and dinner is sufficient.

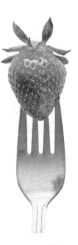

It is surprising how choosing lean, low-fat protein foods at thirty-five to fifty calories per ounce increases satiety and enables an easier way to keep within a calorie goal.

There are circumstances when eating more protein is required, but this is at the other end of the weight spectrum. A large man or overweight or obese woman with a calorie needs between 1,800-2,000 often requires larger protein servings to meet calorie and satiety needs. In this situation use the following guidelines:

3 servings of protein at breakfast
(2 eggs, 1 ounce lean ham)

1 serving mid-morning
(1 ounce low-fat cheese)

6 servings at lunch
(6 ounces turkey)

1–2 serving mid-afternoon
(2 ounces tuna)

6 servings at dinner
(6 ounces chicken)

Quick Protein Calculator

A quick way to calculate how much protein you need is to take your weight in pounds and divide it in half. This number equals the approximate number of grams of protein you should eat each day. A more in-depth analysis of protein goals is dependent on fat allowances which include a number of factors so let's explore fat first.

The Skinny on Fat

I could write an entire book on this misunderstood subject. Just like the diet mentality made us carb phobic, the reports on fats made us shun even the good fats. Even today, every new research report causes a media frenzy. It is enough to make my head spin. I suppose, though, that if you consider that one of the problems with nutrition research results and its incongruities stems from the fact that nutrition was a governmental afterthought until the 1940s when we became concerned about the best way to feed our troops during World War II, then you can understand the emergence of new information as studies are completed. Early on, the field of nutrition had relied mainly on short-term studies, so without adequate time to follow up various findings, it was inevitable that different studies yielded different results. In the 1960s a greater concern arose about our health and even more studies were completed and reported. However, our best answers have come from long-term studies with their large subject populations and adequate time for follow up. So today, if you follow the recent nutrition claims, it does seem like one food or vitamin is harmful one year and not the next. Or you read that eating X will fight disease only to read later that it doesn't. But not so the studies of fats, these have been consistent since the 1960s. So, let's learn how fat impacts your health and your weight.

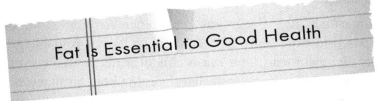

Fat Is Essential to Good Health

Before I give you the scoop on fat and its place in your meal plan, let me emphasize that eating fat is essential to good health. Fats are a necessary component in your body. Fats are present in cell structures and hormones, and they help provide insulation in the form of padding from injury and the cold. Without some fat stores, the body has no backup energy supply. Maybe we are not overly concerned about famine these days or having to hunt for our food, but we do tend to get sick with illnesses that prevent us from eating a sufficient number of calories which in turn uses up reserve fat stores and depletes our bodies even more. Maintaining a healthy amount of body fat is especially important as we get older, and I recommend that people actually aim for a higher percentage of healthy body fat at an advanced age. Recommendations for a healthy percentage of body fat are:

Age	up to 30	30–50	50+
Female	14–21%	15–23%	16–25%
Male	9–15%	11–17%	12–19%

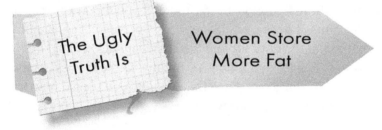

The Ugly Truth Is → Women Store More Fat

I can actually hear the groans. Yes, women are biologically predisposed to store more fat than men, so it's not your imagination. The main reason for this is childbearing. As many women can attest, pregnancy wreaks havoc on the body in many ways, including an increase in body fat that may stay on the hips long after the baby is born. But, losing this baby weight and returning to your normal weight as soon as you can is the course of action that works best to more easily maintain a healthy weight throughout life.

In no way is this easy, but it is absolutely doable. That said, let's get back to fats. What we love about dietary fat is how it enhances the texture of food, adds to the taste, and increases satiety. Dietary fats are also a great source of fat-soluble vitamins A, D, E, and K.

Dietary Fat Makes Body Fat

The connection needs to be made between dietary fat and body fat. Dietary fats, healthy or not, are easily converted to body fat. All dietary fats contain nine calories per gram, whether they are healthy fats or not, more than twice the calories of carbohydrates and proteins (which are each four calories per gram). Fats are a calorie-dense food, which means they impart a large number of calories in very small volume. (A teaspoon of oil or eight nuts yields about forty-five calories, 1/4 cup of nuts equals a whopping 160–180 calories).

High-fat foods need to be eaten in smaller portions to meet calorie needs than low-fat foods. This is why you always need to measure high-fat foods, such as nuts, because it is just too easy to eat too much.

Also remember that low-fat does not mean low-calorie and fat-free does not mean calorie-free and that is why low-fat diet strategies do not lead to weight loss. A common problem in low-fat diets is that we tend to eat, either consciously or unconsciously, larger portions of low-fat foods while wrongly assuming that they are also low calorie. These excess calories are stored as fat and do not ever result in weight loss no matter what their source.

Another problem is that when we think we are making healthy food choices we tend to eat more. This, of course, defeats the purpose. Excess calories are excess calories, but where fats are concerned, there is an added wrinkle in that some are good for us and some are definitely not. Fats are not created equally.

With Saturated Fats Go Slow, Give Trans Fats the Heave-Ho

It has been documented that saturated fats and trans fats lead to heart disease. Since we know that saturated and trans fats increase LDL cholesterol and triglycerides and compromise heart health, it is wise to limit your fat intake as well as be selective as to the types of fats you consume. For example, butter tastes great, but butter is all saturated fat. This means you can still enjoy it if you use less of it. By using less you limit the amount of saturated fat added to that meal. Consider this, there are times you might prefer the taste of a full-fat cheese, such as when you snack on cheese and crackers, but other times, say when you are making chicken parmigiana, you can get away with using a low-fat variety. Better yet, use shredded cheese in cooking so that you can use less but cover more of the food with it. What's more, melted cheese loses its texture, anyway, so why waste the fat grams under those circumstances. Likewise, the fat in mayonnaise is also discretionary. If you are spreading mayo on bread for a turkey sandwich, you may want the taste of the regular full-fat variety, but for tuna salad or in a sauce or dressing, the reduced-fat variety will work just as well because the other ingredients overpower the taste of the mayo anyway. In fact, using reduced-fat mayo three times a week in place of regular can save you 10,000 calories a year. How easy is that?

Monounsaturated and Polyunsaturated, the Healthy Fats

Both the monounsaturated fats found in olive oil, canola oil, and nuts, and the polyunsaturated fats found in vegetable oils, nuts, and fish (commonly known as omega-3 fatty acids) add all heart

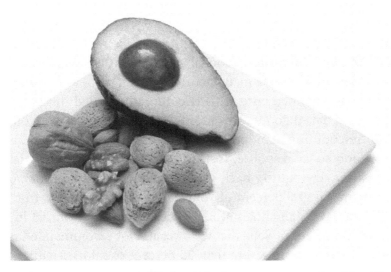

and texture to your food while boosting your health. These healthy fats are also easy to integrate into your diet. The next time you are eating bread with dinner, try dipping it in a flavorful olive oil instead of spreading it with butter. Instead of that pat of butter on your vegetables, sauté them in a little olive oil and garlic. If you think you can't live without the taste of butter, then try one of the excellent tasting butter substitutes on the market. Just be careful not to choose those with trans fats as they are even more harmful to your health than saturated fats. I have experimented with vegan butter substitutes in everything from mashed potatoes to baked goods and my family has raved about the food without knowing I made the switch (I guess they do now).

Make Smart Low-Fat Choices

There are so many low-fat choices today that it's hard to know which products to buy or how to incorporate them into your diet. So let's start with the basics.

Low-fat products, by law, must have three grams or less fat per serving. But low-fat foods often have less taste, so manufacturers make the foods taste better by adding ingredients you need to avoid. So begin by reading food labels to help you avoid another dietary minefield. Some manufacturers add sugar to reduced-fat products to enhance taste. This is common in salad dressings, sauces, and baked goods. This means it is also problematic from a calorie-counting standpoint, carbohydrate-limiting goals, or even blood sugar response. Instead of blindly choosing low-fat alternatives, try cutting back on full-fat foods and aim for no more than 25-30% percent of your daily calories to come from fat. If you have high cholesterol, it is best to modify your fat intake to 25 percent of your diet to lower it. Not recommended is a fat restriction more severe than 25 percent of calories without consulting a Registered Dietitian Nutritionist or other health professional if weight loss is the only goal. For most adults, that translates to forty to sixty grams of fat per day.

Here is how to cut the fat:

1,200 daily calorie goal

30% of 1,200 = 360 calories from fat

360 calories divided by 9 calories per gram = 40 grams of fat/day

1,500 daily calorie goal

30% of 1,500 = 450 calories from fat

450 calories divided by 9 calories per gram = 50 grams of fat/day

1,800 daily calorie goal

30% of 1,800 = 540 calories from fat

540 calories divided by 9 calories per gram = 60 grams of fat/day

No Label? No Problem

It is easy to count grams of fat when they are printed on a food label, but what to do about meat or chicken which don't come with such a label? Well, steak has up to eight grams of fat per ounce. White meat chicken and fish have zero to one gram of fat per ounce. Dark meat poultry, pork, and leaner cuts of beef have about five grams of fat per ounce. This is why it is important to choose animal proteins wisely.

What you put between the bread in a sandwich can add or save a significant number of calories. Three ounces of fresh deli turkey is about 105 calories and little, if any, fat. Three ounces of salami or bologna clock in at 300 calories and twenty-four grams of fat—half the recommended daily amount for many people! If you love salami, sausage, or hot dogs, you needn't stop eating them, but what you do need is to consider them only as a choice for when you want to splurge.

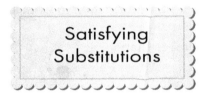

Satisfying
Substitutions

Another tip is to learn to balance out the day's eating when calculating total daily fat intake. By this I mean that when you have a high-fat meal, you balance it out by eating a lower-fat meal in the same day. You can also make lower-fat substitutions for foods like sour cream, cream cheese, crackers, and chips. Do this at every opportunity, be it grocery shopping for home-cooked meals or picking up lunch at the deli.

For breakfast stay away from high-fat fast-food breakfast sandwiches. Try scrambled egg whites or egg substitute on a roll and follow with fresh fruit instead.

For lunch consider a grilled chicken or roasted turkey sandwich, salad, and light dressing instead of a cheeseburger and fries. There are so many healthy choices you can make, and once you get in this frame of mind, you will be able to recognize many more.

For dinner (or all meals) prepare food by baking, grilling, or broiling it, instead of frying. Even pan sautéing and stir-frying are good options because they use only a small amount of oil and the food does not absorb much of it. Substitute an olive oil spray and a nonstick pan to brown food with little fat. Air-fryers have become a popular alternative to frying everything from chicken to kale.

Seriously, by following the above suggestions you may have just found an easy way to eliminate calories and unhealthy fats from your life and not even miss them.

Putting It All Together

It's now time to put this information to work and choose healthy foods.

To begin, remember that:

► *Carbohydrates should be no more than 50 percent of your total calories*

► *Fat intake should represent no more than 30 percent of your total calories*

► *Protein should be 20 percent of your calories*

If you have high cholesterol or triglycerides, it is recommended to reduce your fat and carbohydrate intake resulting in higher protein to meet your calorie needs.

Take note that I am not advocating a high-protein diet, but because the restriction on fat and carbs is necessary for heart health, the sources of calories and food group choices is reduced, which increases the reliance on protein as a calorie source.

Tracking Daily Protein and Fat Intake

To track daily protein and fat intake, you can choose either to count calories or grams/servings.

For Protein: Because protein has four calories per gram, take your protein calorie goal total and divide by four grams. Because there are six to seven grams of protein in most animal protein sources per ounce, divide the grams of protein by seven. Each ounce of fish, chicken, beef, pork, and cheese will be the equivalent of one serving of protein.

For fats: Fats are nine calories per gram. Take the total daily calorie goal for fat and divide by nine to get the number of fat grams per day. You can count grams or servings. There are five grams of fat in one serving of fat. So divide your fat gram goal by five to calculate how many servings of fat you should have each day. Cheese, along with most one-ounce servings of beef, pork, and prepared meats, has one serving of fat. One teaspoon of oil, butter, and regular salad dressing also counts as one serving.

Let's now take a look at what a typical 1,600-calorie diet would include: 800 calories of carbohydrates (50%), 480 calories of fat (30%), and 320 calories of protein (20%). That said, a person with those calorie goals will be including 200 grams of carbohydrates per day, 80 grams of protein, and 53 (53.3 to be exact) grams of fat.

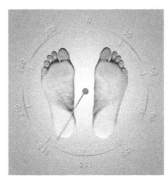

1,200-Calorie Sample One-Day Menu

Breakfast

1 multigrain English muffin
3 egg whites
1/2 cup chopped tomatoes/onions
Olive oil spray

Mid-Morning Snack

Low-fat, low-sugar, yogurt
1/4 cup high-fiber cereal

Lunch

2 slices whole wheat bread
4 ounces turkey breast
Lettuce, tomato, 1 tsp. mustard
6 baby carrots
1 medium pear

Afternoon snack

1 medium apple

Dinner

4 ounces baked chicken with herbs
6 ounces baked sweet potato
1 cup steamed broccoli
1 cup garden salad
2 tbsp. low-fat salad dressing
1 tsp. cooking oil

1,400-Calorie Sample One-Day Menu

Breakfast

1 cup oatmeal with cinnamon
3/4 cup berries
8 ounces nonfat milk

Mid-Morning Snack

1 ounce low-fat cheese
8 wheat thin crackers

Lunch

1 cup low sodium minestrone or bean soup
1 cup garden salad
2 tbsp. low-fat dressing
1 apple

Afternoon snack

1 cup raw vegetables
2 tbsp. hummus

Dinner

4 ounces frozen cooked shrimp
1 1/2 cups frozen stir-fry vegetables
2/3 cup cooked brown rice
2 tsp. cooking oil

Evening snack

8 ounces nonfat milk

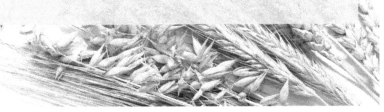

1,600-Calorie Sample One-Day Menu

Breakfast
2 slices whole wheat bread
1 tbsp. peanut butter
1 small banana sliced
1 cup nonfat milk

Mid-Morning Snack
6 ounces nonfat vanilla yogurt
3/4 cup blueberries

Lunch
4 ounces (3/4 cup diced) cooked boneless
    chicken breast
1 cup mixed salad greens
1 cup chopped raw vegetables
1/4 cup chick peas
2 tbsp. dried cranberries
2 tbsp. low-fat ranch dressing

Afternoon Snack
1/2 cup (about 15) grapes
7 whole almonds

Dinner
4 ounces cooked salmon
1/4 cup tomato salsa
1 cup corn
1 cup string beans
6 asparagus spears
2 tsp. olive oil or butter substitute

Evening Snack
3 cups low-fat microwave or air-popped popcorn

2,000-Calorie Sample One-Day Menu

Breakfast
1 cup Kashi cereal
8 ounces nonfat milk
1 cup strawberries

Mid-Morning Snack
1/2 whole wheat pita
1 tbsp. peanut butter
1 small banana sliced

Lunch
1 whole wheat wrap
3 ounces tuna mixed with 1 tbsp. mayonnaise
1 cup spinach, shredded carrots, peppers,
    and tomato mix
6 ounces low-fat yogurt

Afternoon snack
1 low-fat granola bar
8 ounces nonfat milk

Dinner
4 ounces cooked pork chop
1 cup quinoa
2 cups cooked spinach sautéed in 2 tsp. olive oil
    and 1 minced garlic clove

Evening snack
1/2 cup light ice cream

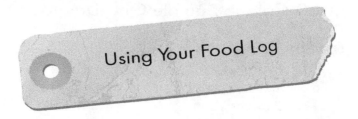

Using Your Food Log

Now take a look at your food journal again. Make note of your protein and fat intake along with your vegetable, fruit, and starch intake. Remember that some foods have more than one nutrient to track and record. For instance, don't forget to count the one serving of protein in your milk/yogurt by marking both milk/yogurt and protein columns, and the beans that count as a serving of starch and a serving of protein. Animal proteins need to be assessed for fat content to improve accuracy of recording. It is more critical that you take notice of whether or not you tend to choose high-fat beef and fast food rather than be concerned with the exact number of grams consumed, so add five grams (or one serving), of fat to the fat column any time you eat those foods if your method of recording does not automatically do it for you. It is more telling to look over the food journal and see, for example, that when the protein column is emptier during the day, it's because you ate too many starches at dinner, or that if you are exceeding your fat allotment, it's because of eating a lot of take-out foods.

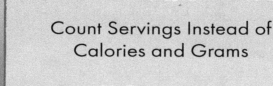

Count Servings Instead of Calories and Grams

Counting servings instead of calories and grams may seem overwhelming at first, but you will find that after a very short time it is an easier way to stick to the goals. As a mathematically challenged individual, I understand that it takes effort to establish target numbers. However, once done, it is easier to look at the number of servings recorded in the journal and see, for instance, you had your two fruits that day but needed to have a yogurt for an evening snack because you didn't drink your milk serving that morning. Or you can quickly evaluate dinner to see that the following day you should have forgone the Italian bread with your pasta because it put you over your starch limit.

As I said before, you can choose to count fat grams, but choosing to count fat servings will make you less likely to miss the added fat servings on the cheeseburger (which comes along with the four servings of protein) at lunch (without the fries) since it didn't come with a label (which, by the way, has twenty-six grams of fat if it came from McDonald's).

Another consideration that makes counting servings easier is that most of us eat the same foods on a regular basis. Think about it. How many different breakfast menus do you actually choose from each morning? Like most of us, it's probably oatmeal one morning and eggs and toast the next. Once you have recorded a menu one time, it is easier to refer back to that entry instead of recalculating another one from scratch. You will probably also have established your portion sizes as well and those entries will also remain fairly constant. It's the same with your other food choices. Again, we tend to be repetitive when it comes to what we eat at lunch and dinner. Snacks, too, are usually another constant. If you aren't a repetitive eater, then by all means find a method or resource that saves you time. If your goal is to keep losing or maintaining weight, do not stop recording your portions and calories in a food journal. Use your food journals to track daily servings of starches, fruits, non-starchy vegetables, milk/yogurt, protein, and fat to insure a healthy, well-balanced diet able to support weight loss. And don't forget to record macronutrient servings to establish the habits that will continue to support weight maintenance.

"After a weight loss of about twenty-five pounds (15 percent of my starting weight), my blood pressure dropped to consistent normal, and my doctor ok'd me going off my blood pressure medication. Using this program was the first time I ever counted calories. Although I usually ate good quality food, I realized I was overeating."

John M.

You are now four weeks in from the start of your journey and you are now following a map with a very clearly detailed route and a defined destination. You are now following a plan that includes specific guidelines on when you eat, how much to eat, and which food groups to choose from. The exact foods you choose to eat are of less consequence if you are burning more calories than you are eating. You now know the importance of eating when hungry and stopping when you have eaten just enough to quell the hunger. You've learned that you can carry snacks on your journey of 100-150 calories each, so you are not overly hungry at meals. To increase your likelihood of success you understand that choosing low-density, highly nutritious foods, including fruits, vegetables, whole grains, and low-fat milk/yogurt and low-fat animal proteins, means consuming a satisfying volume of food with fewer calories. You also know how to plan your plate by being aware of the ratio of carbs, fats, and protein.

You are also balancing your meals so that at day's end, you achieve your calorie and fat goals and reach your recommended servings of protein, vegetables, fruit, milk/yogurt, and starch.

You are also picking up the pace by being able to walk longer, faster, and with more intensity to burn more calories than you were able to do at the outset. You are also now performing aerobic activities that continually challenge your body and will increase your weight loss success.

If at any point in time, your weight loss stops before you are ready to begin weight maintenance, then return to the beginning of this chapter and reassess your goals and your determination to comply with the program and you will succeed. Next try recalculating your calorie needs, as you did in week three (this number does change with significant weight loss) and the subsequent breakdown of macronutrients and recommended servings. It is important to be honest in your assessment of your physical activity since it is an integral factor in weight loss.

Now that you are comfortable on this road to weight loss, it's time to consider the tools and techniques that will keep you from veering off this path to wellness. The plan you are currently following won't change, but your awareness of your environment, how you make food choices, and your food behaviors will.

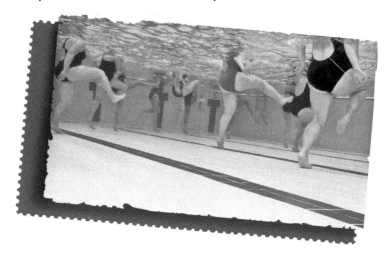

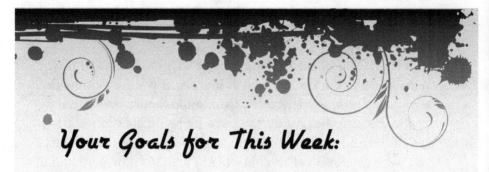

Your Goals for This Week:

1. Continue to keep accurate food journals for accountability and to highlight successes

    a. *Establish appropriate protein, carbohydrate, and fat intake guidelines in number of calories, number of grams, or number of servings*

2. Make intelligent food choices

    a. *Practice Planning the Plate to make it easier to eat the proper ratio of foods at every meal*

    b. *Choose low-density foods*

    c. *Substitute good fat choices for bad ones*

    d. *Make use of the hunger/fullness scale*

3. Try to meet or exceed your planned exercise goal.

    a. *Use the activity tracker to check if you achieved walking 10,000 steps each day*

    b. *Evaluate the frequency, duration, and intensity of your exercise sessions and look for ways to increase all three factors*

4. Keep to your daily calorie goal

    a. *Keep to your daily carbohydrate goal*

    b. *Keep to your daily protein and fat goal*

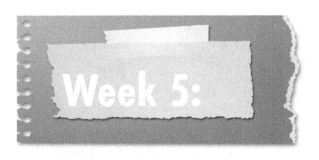

Mindful Eating

Mindful eating is having an awareness of the what, when, where, why, and how we consume food. In today's society, work, family, scheduling pressures, and other extrinsic factors have made highly processed food the acceptable norm for most meals eaten quickly, which makes practicing mindful eating challenging. Take fast food for example. It's not only driving through a fast-food window that makes this type of eating experience fast because fast food can also be the sandwich you scarfed down at your desk in order to meet that deadline at work, or the bowl of cereal you inhaled over the kitchen sink this morning. You see it's not only the way food is prepared and delivered to us fast that we refer to as fast, but also the way in which we eat it that classifies it as a fast-food experience.

Finding Pleasure in Eating

When we eat fast or with distractions, we cannot possibly be present in the full experience of eating, which entails being able to enjoy the taste and texture of the food, assess hunger and fullness level, and find pleasure in the eating experience itself. Simply taking the time to smell your food has a tremendous influence on how quickly your appetite is satisfied. So in addition to bringing home the bacon, it is important to your girth to take time to pause and smell it too. Most of us occasionally dine, but what we are mostly guilty of is eating out of necessity. Any mealtime that places convenience over quality (saving time by multitasking) like entertaining or doing business during a meal, helps to unwittingly pack on the pounds. Those among us at a healthy weight tend to take the time to plan for and prepare meals at home and to set aside the time to enjoy those meals. The people who do this are mindful eaters who remove distractions from mealtime except for pleasant conversations with family or dining mates.[13]

The good news is that you are already on your way to becoming a mindful eater by recording what you have been eating. This simple act means you are paying attention to what, when, why, where and how you eat. I am especially pleased when the people who have lost weight tell me that this method is also a great deterrent to making poor food choices.

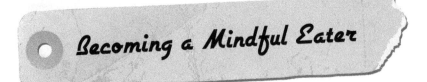

Becoming a Mindful Eater

The following are ways to help you become a mindful eater:

- ► *Be aware of and follow hunger and fullness cues.*

- ► *Pay attention to the grumbling coming from your stomach or the 4 p.m. energy slump.*

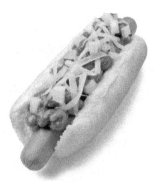

- ► *Use snacks to prevent extreme hunger which helps control how much you eat at meals and reduces binge eating behaviors.*

- ► *Make eating an activity in and of itself. It's true that we tend to eat more while watching TV or when we associate an activity with food—think hot dogs, peanuts, and cotton candy at the ballgame or the bowl of ice cream while watching the evening news.*

- ► *Plate your food from the stove or counter and don't put s erving bowls on the table. We tend to eat more food when we can see it, so leave temptation in the kitchen.*

- ► *Eat slowly, take smaller bites, chew your food longer, put the fork down between bites*

External cues and the environment can stimulate or encourage eating more. Large plates, drinking glasses, food containers influence how much we eat and drink. That's why it's best to eat measured portions from a plate, bowl, or snack-size bag instead of eating directly from a large package or container. Brian Wansink's study of moviegoers eating popcorn found that the larger the container the more popcorn was eaten—even when the popcorn was stale.[14] Likewise, this research also showed that the size of the plates and bowls influenced how much his subjects ate. So before you start eating, divide the contents of large containers into single servings or portions (this also goes for food in take-out containers) and eat from small plates and bowls.

Taking the ≡ FAST Out of Fast Food

The speed at which we eat is a major reason for weight gain. It takes twenty minutes for your stomach to tell your brain that you have had enough. When we eat fast because we are overly hungry or pressed for time, it renders this crucial stomach-to-brain message impossible.

In order to keep the lines of this brain/stomach communication open and keep yourself from eating extra calories, eat slowly, take smaller portions, and always wait a few minutes before taking a second helping to give your brain time to acknowledge when your hunger is satisfied. If later you find that you still feel hungry, you can snack. This simple action will stop you from eating to the point of being overly full.

Nothing takes the fast out of fast food like slowing down. You may find you need to do this by putting your fork or spoon down between bites and making sure to thoroughly chew and swallow before taking the next bite. Taking a sip water between bites also helps to slow the eating process. Choose the strategy that works best for you. Also try setting a timer for twenty-minutes at the beginning of the meal so you won't refill your plate until it goes off. This allows you to know for sure whether or not you are truly satisfied or really do need to eat more. This is yet another reason to plate your food at the stove or counter because if you want more you'll have to physically get up and go get it. This very act will give you time to ask yourself, "Am I still hungry?"

Don't clear the table so fast. Leave empty plates and wrappers in plain sight as a reminder of the amount of food you've eaten or splurged. Empty wrappers keep us honest. A study on food amnesia by Brian Wansink found when chicken wing bones were cleared from the table diners underestimated how much they ate by 50 percent. [15]

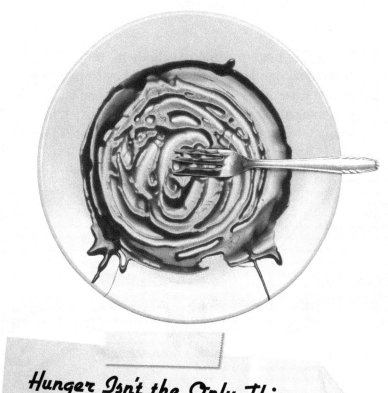

Hunger Isn't the Only Thing That Makes Us Eat

Hunger, like all human behavior, is driven by external and internal factors. These factors are called antecedents and are the events, situations, and emotions that precede any behavior, emotion, or action. An antecedent is also an eating trigger that can be controlled or removed from your environment. Once it's removed or altered, a behavior can be changed and any unwanted consequences, such as overeating and regret, are avoided. This sequence of events is called a "behavior chain" and here's how it works.

Jane was tired after a long day so she had settled down on the couch to watch TV. During a commercial for Dunkin' Donuts, she went to the kitchen cabinet where she took out the package of chocolate chip cookies and brought it back to the couch where she sat with it in her lap while she ate them. It was only at the next commercial that Jane realized she had eaten half the package. This made her angry with feelings of regret and guilt because she had sabotaged her weight loss efforts. She also felt full, but it wasn't enough to stop her from finishing off the entire package.

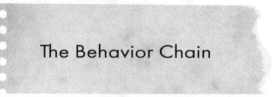

The Behavior Chain

SAMPLE CHAIN

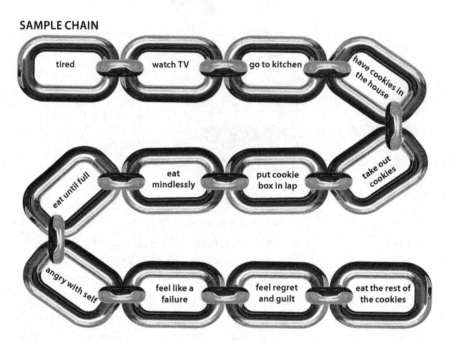

tired — watch TV — go to kitchen — have cookies in the house — take out cookies — put cookie box in lap — eat mindlessly — eat until full — angry with self — feel like a failure — feel regret and guilt — eat the rest of the cookies

In Jane's case, her antecedents were that she was tired, she saw the food, she ate from the package, and she held the package while eating from it. This was pure mindless eating because Jane had not only not taken the time to pay attention to the taste, but she also didn't practice portion control. Jane's consequence for this action resulted in her consuming many more calories than was appropriate, feeling uncomfortable, and being upset with herself. This was further followed with more negative thoughts and an attitude that in turn led to eating even more cookies. We could take this behavior chain even further by adding more antecedents like the fact that the cookies were even in the house or why she chose that particular time to eat them.

In order to understand how certain behaviors in your life link together to trigger eating, create your own chain of events and behaviors based on your past experiences of mindless eating and the remorse you felt afterward. Keep in mind that your reasons or circumstances may paint a completely different scenario than Jane's. Try to be as specific in the details as you can in recalling this event.

Finding the Weakest Link

Many antecedent events are really lapses or errors in judgment. They are based more on habit than active decision-making and not weakness or lack of willpower. This means that you can stop an event from repeating itself by identifying and changing the behavior early on. This is akin to breaking the weakest link in the behavior chain. Listed below is a breakdown as to how Jane could have done things differently to break the link in her chain:

- ▶ *Not kept the cookies in the house*

- ▶ *Taken only two cookies and put them on a plate then placed the plate on the coffee table*

- ▶ *Broken each cookie into four pieces and eaten only one piece at a time, being careful not to eat another piece until all the cookie taste was gone from her palate*

- ► Chosen a snack-size bag of microwave popcorn instead
- ► Eaten slowly to taste each piece of cookie therefore being alert to fullness cues
- ► Acknowledged how good the snack tasted

Your Chain

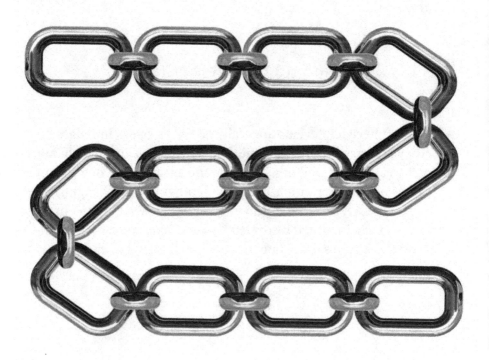

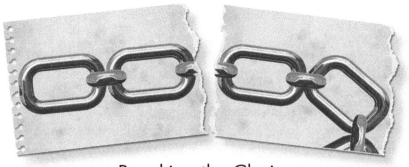

Breaking the Chain

The first step in breaking the chain is to identify the triggers or problem situations, environments, or activities that lead to inappropriate eating. Below is a checklist to start you off with blank spaces provided for you to add your own triggers.

Seeing food

Smelling food

Cooking food

Sitting at the computer

Watching TV

Celebrating holiday

Being tired

Being bored

Feeling anxious

Being with certain people

Talking on the phone

Attending a party or gathering

Being at work

Feeling happy

Feeling angry

Feeling deserving of a reward

Being on vacation

Drinking alcohol

Ending the day

Being sad/hurt/upset

_____

_____

_____

_____

Doing this exercise led one of my clients to avoid the places in her house where she kept food after she had eaten her evening snack. Instead, she prepared for bedtime and read in bed for an hour before falling asleep. Not only did her new behavior cut down on night-time eating, but she found she was falling asleep easier, sleeping longer, and eating less the next day because she was not sleep deprived. Another client found that instead of just sitting down and eating his evening snack, he took the time to arrange his chips and salsa on a plate as if he were serving a guest. In doing this, he found that a smaller portion was even more satisfying. The simple act of presentation made all the difference.

In thinking through the triggers and food behaviors that lead to choosing unhealthy foods and/or eating without attending to fullness cues helps us to better understand this unhealthy habit. This understanding is what leads to making a successful plan of action based on healthy decision making. Practicing the plan replaces the unhealthy behaviors and over time establishes a new healthier habit—with a positive outcome all around.

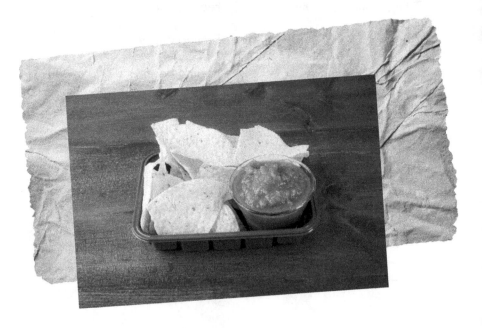

"I am four pounds away from the twenty-five pounds I have been fighting with for years! Because of my current successful weight loss, I was able to qualify for a lower rate for my life insurance policy. It was most beneficial for me to keep food out of sight (off the counters) as it was much easier to not think of food if I didn't see it. Today I also don't eat the next bite until I can no longer taste the last one. I've learned that the longer it takes to eat gives your brain the time it needs to register how full I am."

Steven

Junk Food and Emotional Eating

Mindless eating and binge eating are often emotionally driven responses which makes it easier to focus on the good food/bad food conundrum instead of addressing the use of food to soothe or reward.

No food is bad. Junk food refers to foods that are of lower nutrition quality. Yes, there are better food choices, healthier options, or better portion sizes, but no food is bad. We do think of chips, sweets, and high-fat foods as bad which creates a dilemma since we are genetically programmed to favor high-fat and high-sugar foods. When you think of a food as forbidden, you will either choose that food when you feel deserving of a reward or feel guilt and remorse when you eat it, both of which lead to an unhealthy eating event.

Learning to allow yourself a food that is high in sugar, fat, or both, without guilt when you want it, means the amount you eat becomes less important. For example, if you only allow yourself ice cream when you are feeling sad, you will tend to eat the whole pint, probably mindlessly, while distracting yourself with a movie or streaming your favorite series. Instead, try eating a half a cup (in a small dish) of the low-fat variety as a snack when you want. I am a chocoholic and I know that if I deprive myself of chocolate day in and day out that when I do have the opportunity to indulge (like when my accountant leaves a box of Godiva on my desk each December), I will probably eat more of it than I would if I allowed myself the occasional piece. (Oh let's be real, without my chocolate fix, I would eat the entire box at one sitting). To prevent this type of behavior, I have an appropriate portion of chocolate once a day on the days I feel like it. I say once a day because that is how I can be sure that this low-nutrient snack is not replacing the healthier snack foods in my diet, such as fruit. I prefer my chocolate in the evening, which means if you offer me cake or cookies midday I will decline since my once-a-day rule means I would have to forgo my evening chocolate. If I do indulge in mid-afternoon birthday cake, I reach for the fruit that evening that would have been my afternoon snack and skip the chocolate. Since I also follow the 100- to 150-calorie snack rule, I have my options already planned. If your thing is chips, figure out what kind and how many chips satisfy you and eat only that amount. If you are not sure of your ability to portion control at any given moment, break down the larger bag into portion sizes as soon as you get home from the store.

The Rule of Healthy Snacking

The rule is: Eat what you really enjoy but eat it mindfully. You need to eat slowly to be mindful of the taste and texture of every bite and how good it makes you feel to eat it. For cookies or chocolate, prepare to eat them in small bites. Break cookies and chocolate into small pieces and put them on a plate. Take the first piece and then move the plate just out of reach. Savor that bite and do not take another piece until you can no longer taste the first one. Not only does this cause you to be more mindful of each bite, but the eating event will be longer and more satisfying because you will have tasted each and every bite. Compare eating in this way to sitting down with a handful of cookies and having them eaten before you actually register their taste in your mouth. In reality, you do not actually enjoy subsequent pieces of a sweet as much as you enjoy the first one or two bites. If you are eating sweets in a mindful way, I can guarantee that you will be satisfied with smaller portions than you are used to.

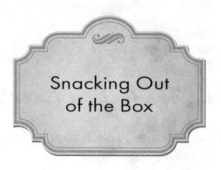

Snacking Out of the Box

For many of us, our snack choices are driven by convenience. Whether at our desk, in the car, or at home, with some thought and planning, snacks can provide opportunities to not only control our hunger but improve our nutrition status. Between meal snacks should include food groups that may be lacking or missing from your breakfast, lunch, and dinner. For example, if you do not typically include a fruit at meals, use fruit as between meal snacks to insure you get your two to four servings in every day. If your calcium-rich food intake is low, grab low-fat yogurt for a midday boost.

Many foods are prepackaged making them easy and quick but not very nutritious. There are many ways to improve the nutrient content of snacks we typically find in containers. Add an ounce of low-fat cheese to whole grain crackers. Mix almonds and raisins with pretzel goldfish. Enjoy eight ounces of nonfat milk with one multigrain or buttermilk frozen waffle.

Fruit is an easy grab and go snack. Increase your satiety and protein intake by adding an ounce of low-fat cheese to your apple or spread a measured tablespoon of peanut butter on your banana. Mix a cup of strawberries or blueberries with plain or vanilla nonfat yogurt. Fruit could be your new choice in "fast" food.

What about when you have the time or interest in getting out of the box. Here are some new snack suggestions to get you thinking and wake up the taste buds while providing health-boosting nutrients.

1/2 English muffin, 1 ounce 2 percent milk cheese, 1 tomato slice

1 ounce sliced turkey wrapped around 1 low-fat cheese stick

1 ounce part skim mozzarella, 2 slices tomato, 1 slice roasted red pepper optional

1 cup Campbell's Select Harvest light soup, 5 wheat thins

1/2 cup low-fat cottage cheese, 1/2 cup berries

2 ounces tuna packed in water, 5 saltine crackers

3 shrimp, 1 tbsp. cocktail sauce

2 ounces sliced turkey/ romaine lettuce rollups

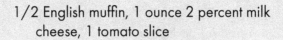

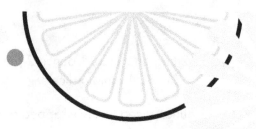

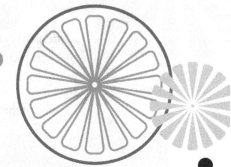

1 mini pita, 1 tbsp.
   hummus, chopped
   cucumber and tomato

2 tbsp. chopped avocado,
   2 tbsp. chopped tomato,
   7 corn tortilla chips

1 small pear, 1 ounce shaved aged asiago
   or parmesan cheese

1/2 slice dense multigrain bread, 2 tsp. goat cheese,
   3 strawberries sliced, 1/2 tsp. honey

3 oz. baked potato with salsa or fat-free sour cream
   on top

2 tsp. peanut butter spread over a frozen banana

1/2 cup frozen edamame, cooked according to pkg.
   directions, lightly salted

1/2 cup bean salad, jarred or homemade

Snacks 100 Calories or Less

1 Jolly Time Healthy Pop 100 calorie mini bag popcorn

40 Rold Gold Classic Style Pretzel sticks

1 Yoplait light smoothie

1/2 cup low-fat cottage cheese with 5 strawberries

25 grapes

1/2 medium cantaloupe

1/2 red bell pepper dipped in 3 tbsp. hummus

1 slice tomato with 1/2 ounce part-skim mozzarella cheese

2 tsp. peanut butter on 1 slice light whole wheat toast

2 Eggo mini waffles with 1 tsp. syrup

29 Pistachios

15 baby carrots with 2 tbsp. low-fat dressing

5 Nabisco Nilla Wafers

1 Healthy Choice Mocha Fudge Swirl Bar

9 mini Tootsie Rolls

1 Skinny Cow fat-free fudge bar

1 Nestle Butterfinger Stixx

1 Vitamuffin Vitatop

60 Pepperidge Farm Baby Goldfish crackers

Campbell's soup on hand, e.g., blended
     vegetable medley

1/2 mini bagel with 1 ounce smoked salmon

2 cups raspberries

1 cup blueberries

15 strawberries dipped in 1/4 cup CoolWhip lite

2 tbsp. avocado and 2 tbsp. tomato in half mini pita

1 fat-free pudding cup

1 cup romaine with
     2 tbsp. low-fat
     Caesar dressing

8 peanut butter Ritz Bits

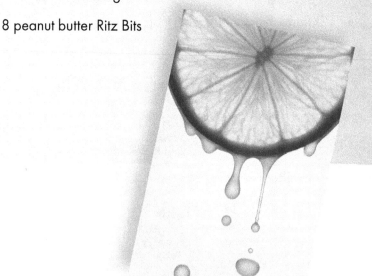

Eat What You Like

Eliminating any one food or food group does not necessarily help you lose weight. In fact restriction and deprivation can cause just the opposite. Knowing how to eat—not fad dieting—is what causes weight loss. Stop following the mass-produced one-diet-fits-all approach. Instead, take small steps, practice new behaviors until they feel comfortable and become easier, maybe even effortless. Become a mindful eater.

When you become a mindful eater you make the change from eating out of habit to becoming an active decision maker by choosing healthy foods you will enjoy. Start with foods like yogurt, in your favorite flavor, as a dessert, or raw vegetables dipped in Ranch dressing instead of potato chips and onion dip. This is the time to seek out new foods to replace unhealthy choices or even to experiment with new ways to prepare your favorite foods. Instead of boring steamed broccoli, roast it in the oven tossed with olive oil and salt. Replace fatty cheese and sugary ketchup on your burger with flavorful, nutrient-packed, low-calorie sauteed mushrooms and onions. Swap your next beef burger with a turkey or salmon burger. And if you slip and forget to measure that portion of fries, don't beat yourself up, just remember the next time. It's all about being honest with yourself and acknowledging that you could have chosen better. Then follow up with planning out a better way to cope in future situations where you are confronted with tempting foods. These are all ways to turn any poor choice into a learning experience and allow you to feel good about how you handled the consequences. Above all, never try to revamp your entire diet overnight. Instead, strive to accomplish small changes which will reward you with increasing your confidence. Each successful food decision will encourage you to make yet another positive change. And if you have one of those days when nothing but a cheeseburger will satisfy you, then go for it and reward yourself.

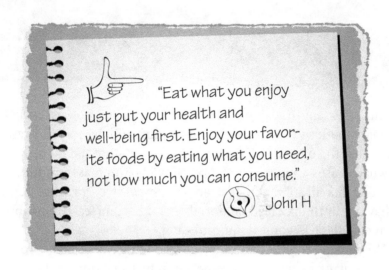

"Eat what you enjoy just put your health and well-being first. Enjoy your favorite foods by eating what you need, not how much you can consume."

John H

Portion Distortion

Another factor that influences and sometimes confuses how much we need to eat is determining correct portion size. Most packaged foods come with a printed nutrition label suggesting serving size but often that suggested serving size, say two cups of cooked pasta or a typical bagel, may not be right for everyone, especially for those of us struggling with weight. Equating those portions to 6 slices and 4 slices of bread, respectively, may illustrate why to you need to rethink portion sizes. Granted, it is difficult to avoid overeating when many high-calorie food come in such large packaging and the serving size is chosen by the food company and is based on what today's average consumer eats—which tends to be a large portion. Following that serving size will influence you to perhaps eat more than you need. The following list shows how serving sizes have changed over the past twenty years:

Bagel   *20 years ago 3-inch diameter, 140 calories*
                     Today 6-inch diameter 350, calories

French fries   *20 years ago 2.4 oz., 210 calories*
                     Today 6.9 oz., 610 calories

Soda   *20 years ago 6.5 oz., 85 calories*
                     Today 20 oz., 165 calories

**Turkey
Sandwich**   *20 years ago 320 calories*
                     Today 820 calories

Muffin   *20 years ago 210 calories*
                     Today 500 calories

Saving and Spending the Money in Your Calorie Wallet

My clients really identify with daily calories being compared to money in a wallet because it's just like having a set amount of money to spend each day. Here's how to do this yourself: Start by deciding how you are going to budget the day. With money we determine what we intend to pay for gas, childcare, and groceries. And if you are like me, I always set aside a little more for incidentals—say just in case I get an invite to the movies. But in this case we're spending calories as we would money. First eat the right amount of vegetables, fruits, whole grains, and low-fat milk/yogurt. Then, if it appeals to you, plan on saving one hundred calories for incidentals or splurge foods each day.

I recently listened to my daughter and her friend making plans for an upcoming vacation to California. As they set their budget breakdown for hotel, rental car, food, and entertainment, they questioned whether they had enough money for both the sunset sail and the tour of the Napa Valley. This sounded to me just like a calorie budget, except instead of counting money we count calories and replace dollars and cents with starches, fruit, and protein. Instead of choosing between a sail or a tour, the decision is to choose between steak or chicken and whether or not to have a glass of wine instead of dessert.

I like shoes, lots of them as a matter of fact. When I am at the mall with a friend, it is unlikely I will be interested in blouses, skirts, or sunglasses because I will be saving my money in case I see a great pair of shoes. I am pretty much the same way with food. I know my sweet tooth. Most days I'm satisfied with a 100-calorie, luxurious sweet snack as my splurge. I find chocolate the most satisfying treat of all, which means that when a great chocolate opportunity comes along (for me that is warm molten chocolate cake) I will guiltlessly splurge on the calories. The thing is I am not tempted by cheesecake, carrot cake, or vanilla ice cream because I am saving the calories in my calorie budget for the thing I enjoy the most because it will satisfy me the most. If you do the same, like me you'll be able to enjoy your splurges free from guilt and added pounds.

The idea of spending your calories should help you if you are regularly over your daily calorie goal (think calorie budget). This technique is also useful if you are looking for a way to add back the cheese on your sandwich at lunch or the cookie you used to eat after dinner. Most plans, even those as low as 1,200 calories, have room for a hundred luxury calories after all the healthy fixed "expenses" like vegetables, fruits, whole grains, and low-fat dairy are accounted for.

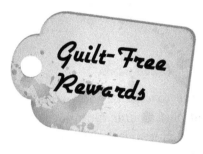

Guilt-Free Rewards

Enjoying a treat helps us not only feel cared-for and content, but also gives us the wherewithal to continue with healthy behaviors. By connecting positive emotions to healthier food choices and meeting exercise goals, we increase the likelihood of choosing good behavior again and again. Using a system of rewards in place of food to celebrate, soothe, or de-stress is an important part of mindfulness. These rewards can be tangible, such as a massage, new kitchen gadget, or a ticket to a sporting event, or as intangible as taking time to leisurely read the Sunday paper or take a bath. If I am stressed at the end of my day or when I complete a project, my reward is to phone my family and tell them I will be a little late so I can stop by the bookstore. I usually don't purchase anything, but this treat makes me feel calm and helps me empty my mind. It piques my interest, my curiosity, and feelings of contentment. And I don't need to spend a dime.

In addition, rewards also function as a positive influence in choosing smaller portion sizes. One study led by Martin Reinmann at the University of Arizona, Leveraging the Happy Meal Effect, showed that pairing a smaller portion of pizza and burgers with a non-food prize was favored by both adults and children over the larger serving with no prize, providing evidence that

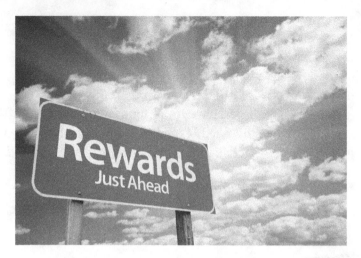

non-food rewards motivate people to change food behaviors. Also noteworthy was the fact that participants did not eat more at subsequent meals to make up for choosing the smaller meal.

There are lots of ways to reward yourself besides food, which has only become a habit. Start with a list of things you like and activities you enjoy. Rewarding short-term efforts pays off in long-term success so you may want to save up for something big. I had one client who had difficulty sticking to her walking plan, so she put a dollar in a jar each day she completed her walking goal to save up for the reflexology she always wanted. Another client rewarded herself for eating mindfully with curling up in her favorite chair with a book. You can make this work for you, too, and all you need to do is to use your good behaviors to achieve a big reward, with the added bonus of making it easier to get to a healthy weight.

Another good idea is to take the money you normally spend on soda or ice cream and use it for an exercise class or use what you save on fast-food lunches toward a new bicycle. Think, too, about the new clothes you are going to need. You are working hard, go ahead, you deserve a reward.

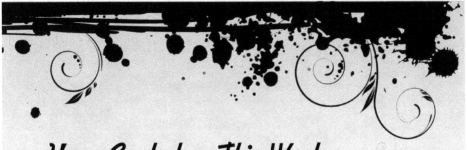

Your Goals for This Week:

1. Remain diligent. Keep measuring food portions, recording everything you eat and drink, and monitoring calorie and carbohydrate intake to meet chosen goals

2. Continue to practice mindful eating behavior.

3. Construct a behavior chain for a challenging situation or an eating event you would like to change

4. Identify antecedents in your life and an environmental and behavioral change you will practice this week to affect the outcome in a new way

5. Decide if you need a reward system in place to succeed in your goals and take the necessary steps to comply with the terms of the reward and toward earning it

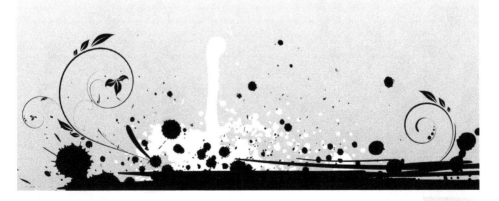

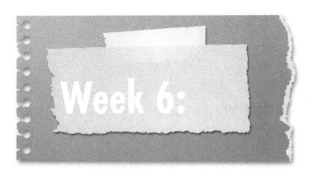

Week 6:

Releasing Your Inner Chef

After all this talk about eating right, it's time to address how to make these foods available and convenient. In order to eat healthier, you need to be able to prepare healthy meals instead of relying on fast and prepared foods. You also need healthy snacks at hand at school, the office, the car, etc., so you can skip the trip to the 7–11 and feed money into vending machines. The first step is to cook your own food, so you first need to get into the habit of going food shopping and doing it well. So let's start by making sure you know how to read a food label.

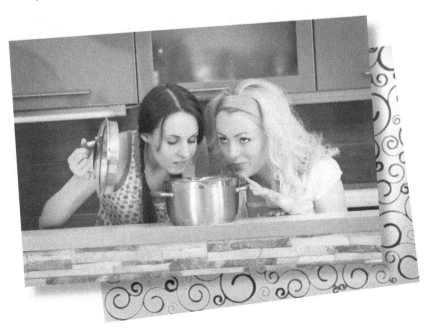

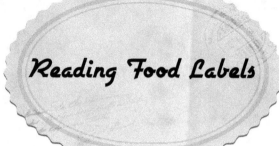

Reading Food Labels

Our sample label is one typically found on a box of breakfast cereal. I chose this type of food label as an example, but I also want you to check out the labels on the foods you have in your kitchen to help you get familiar and secure with what you need to know when making food-buying decisions. Having this knowledge will also speed up your shopping experience, important for those of us who are tight on time or short on patience.

The List of Ingredients

All the ingredients in the package are listed starting with the ingredient present in the largest quantity.

Whole grains, vegetables, fruits, and low-fat dairy products should be listed first on the label of most, if not all, the foods you eat. When the first few ingredients listed are processed flour and sugar, reconsider this food choice.

Fats listed as vegetable, olive, and canola oils are always the fats of choice above butter and any form of hydrogenated oils.

As a general rule, think twice about buying (or eating) any food with an ingredient list that is a paragraph long or contains ingredients you have trouble pronouncing.

The cereal on our sample label gets high marks for having whole wheat, raisins, and wheat bran listed as its first three ingredients. Unfortunately, this wonderful start may be influenced by the next two ingredients, sweeteners, which may influence the decision about whether or not to choose this cereal.

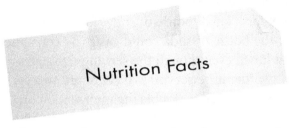

Nutrition facts are always arranged in the same order with the same categories no matter what the food. The comparisons made in terms of percentages are called the percent daily value and are always based on a 2000-calorie diet, which may or not be identical to your calorie needs. This also goes for your sodium or calcium needs which may not be the same as those on which the percentages were based. For our current purposes of learning to read a label, you can set your own needs aside.

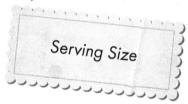

Serving size is important because all the information in the Nutrition Facts is based on it. An important fact to know is that serving size is not based on any industry standard, an American Dietetic Association standard, or anything from the Food and Drug Administration of the United States. It's the manufacturer who determines the serving size of their products.

In order to decide what amount of a particular food is appropriate for you or for an eating event, you may need to multiply, add to, or subtract from the information provided or to get accurate nutrition facts on your portion size. Our sample cereal label states the serving size as one cup. If you find that you need one-and-a-half cups of cereal in the morning, simply calculate what an additional half serving would add to the nutrition facts.

Next, look at the number of servings per container. On a box of breakfast cereal, this probably won't factor into your decision on whether to buy or eat it, but it will for some foods. Check out the label for a small bottle of soda, for instance. The entire contents of the bottle of soda could easily be consumed with a sandwich at lunch even though the serving size states one bottle is equal to two or more servings. If there are two servings per container, you will need to double the information on the label if you plan to drink the entire bottle yourself. Some labels do provide additional information by listing the nutrition facts both by serving size and the entire package.

When you know your portion size and can calculate the nutrition information you are ready to consider the calories per serving.

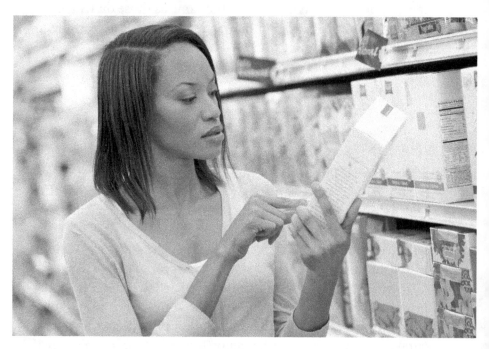

Calories per Serving

You have two decisions to make before you choose this food:

1. Does this product fit into your calorie needs?

2. Will the volume or calorie density (calories to grams) be satisfying?

3. If both answers are yes, continue. If one answer is no, consider whether you want to adjust your portion size to better meet your needs or choose another product. For this cereal, the total calories are more than three times the number of grams per serving, so portions should be limited.

Fat

For fat, apply the same two questions as you did above for calories. To determine fat content either consider the number of calories from fat or the grams of fat, depending on the method you previously chose to monitor your fat intake. For example, this product gets 9 of its 190 calories from fat. On a 1500-calorie diet at 25 percent of the calories from fat, this is 9 out of a daily 375 calories from fat, a fairly low contribution. That translates to forty-one grams of total fat intake for the day (if you are counting fat grams). One gram of total fat in this product reflects a low-fat food and would leave most of your fat allotment for the day to use on other food choices. If one of your health goals is to reduce fat for heart health, lower cholesterol, or to monitor fat intake for weight control, using a low-fat or fat-free milk with this cereal would be a good choice.

The type of fast is the next important fact to glean from any label since saturated fat and trans fats are, as you know, heart health demons. An added bonus for this product is that it is both saturated and trans fat-free. This cereal is also cholesterol-free, which is important to note for heart health.

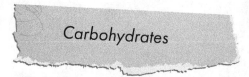

Carbohydrates

The next important nutrition fact listed concerns carbohydrate content. For the purposes of weight loss, and possibly blood sugar control for some of you, remember that we are not looking for foods low in carbohydrates but for foods with complex carbs (which still need to be eaten in moderation). Here, there are forty-seven grams of carbs which is the equivalent of three carb servings (the same as three slices of bread or one cup of pasta). With seven grams of fiber, this product is a good food choice on a high-fiber diet and the fiber content will increase feelings of fullness. The seventeen grams of total sugar include nine grams of added sugar and may not be appropriate for those who prefer a breakfast cereal with less sugar. Without careful consideration, the carbs in high-sugar breakfast foods can closely rival those in some desserts.

Protein

The five grams of protein is approximately one serving of protein which is enough to increase your feeling of fullness as well as your alertness. As such, protein is an important factor to consider when choosing a breakfast food. Along with the milk serving, adding one to two protein servings will complete a well-planned breakfast plate.

Sodium

For heart health and maintaining a healthy blood pressure, always check the sodium content. Base your decision on whether or not to choose a particular food by following the current sodium recommendations of eating less than 2400 mg of sodium/day or 1500 mg/day limit if you have high blood pressure. Because we cannot accurately account for all the salt present in our diet, it is always a good idea to set a lower limit for yourself than you may require. Remember, the only amount of sodium you can accurately account for in your diet is printed on food labels.

In summary, one cup of this cereal along with six ounces of nonfat milk provides two starch servings, one milk serving, one fruit serving, two protein servings, and 250 calories. In addition, its seven grams of fiber make this a good breakfast option in spite of its high sugar content. You decide.

The Shopping Experience

Food shopping does take a bit longer when you start reading food labels, but this is only temporary. But because we tend to purchase many of the same brands and items from week to week, you'll quickly become familiar with the labels on foods you buy often. It took me a while to find the canned tomato products that were the lowest in sodium, but now I am able to quickly reach for the same brand every time, although I do sometimes check to make sure sodium content hasn't changed. I always read the food labels on potentially high-fat items and their lower fat counterparts, like cheeses and condiments, so I make a thoroughly informed decision on how I want to spend my fat calories and the types of fats I consume, especially when it comes to foods I purchase less often.

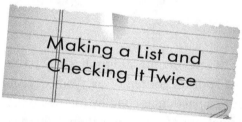

Making a List and Checking It Twice

Shopping from a list is essential so that you do not have to rely on what you need from memory and so you don't impulsively buy the foods you shouldn't be eating. Making a shopping list also helps you to never run out of fruits, vegetables, breakfast items, and healthy snacks which need to be bought frequently. Remember, too, that having a variety of healthy snack choices is key to avoiding the vending machine or cookie cabinet. The person in the household who shops for and prepares the food has 70 percent of the input into what every family member eats. If you don't buy less healthy or high-calorie foods, no one will be tempted to indulge, and not giving into temptation is a main factor in controlling weight. Do this and you will improve the environment for yourself and those you care about, the main factor in overweight.

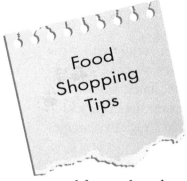

Food Shopping Tips

Keep your shopping list easily accessible so that everyone in your household can add to it, no matter if you do it on paper or electronically. This will make your life simpler. If you are old-school, keep a pad of paper in the kitchen and in the car to make it easy to jot down items you need for meals and snacks as they come to mind. If you are adept at using electronic devices, check out the many apps designed specifically to make food shopping easy. Apps such as Any List or Our Groceries are designed so that others in your household can also download it and add their requests. Other apps such as Paprika, Mealtime and Pepperplate also provide recipes to make meal planning and food shopping easier. With List Ease you list the foods you typically stock in your pantry as well as your next shopping list. The bonus here is keeping better track of your groceries and reducing food waste. Many supermarket chains also have dedicated apps for creating general shopping lists as well as the bonus of linking sale products and electronically downloading coupons for easy checkout.

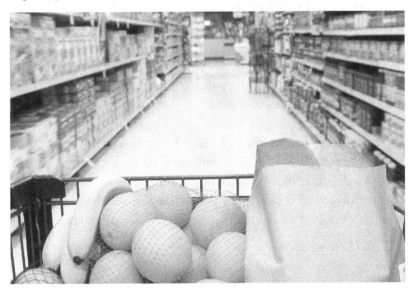

Itemize your groceries in separate columns under either the aisle number or department where they are shelved. For example, make separate columns for produce, dairy, cereals and breads, canned goods, etc. This way you'll save time by picking up like items all at once without having to backtrack in search of forgotten items.

Avoid as many prepared and convenience foods as possible with the exception of ready-to-eat vegetables and fruits. Having these on hand increases the likelihood you will eat them and they make perfect grab-and-go snacks and lunch add-ons. Other healthy convenience foods include canned beans (faster to prepare than dried beans) and quick-cooking grains such as oatmeal and rice.

Stick to buying whole foods and avoid processed ones, including juices, because they provide more nutrients and fewer calories. This means eating an orange rather than drinking orange juice and eating apples more often than apple sauce.

Never shop when hungry or eat food from your shopping cart and you will be better able to resist the temptations lurking on the supermarket shelves.

Shop the walls. The healthiest foods can be found around the perimeter of the store with most prepared and convenience foods in the center aisles.

Go directly from the produce to the fish counter to the poultry to the dairy and only venture down the middle aisles for grains and frozen vegetables.

Park your shopping cart at the end of each aisle. Not only does this increases the number of steps you must take to complete your shopping, because you will need to make trips back and forth to the cart since you can only carry so much in your arms, this technique also decreases your chances of being tempted to spontaneously toss unhealthy, or high calorie, purchases into your cart.

Food Storage Tips

Break down the contents of all food you bring into the house into single serving zip seal food-storage bags or small plastic containers. Making your own pre-portioned snack bags helps with portion control of calorie dense foods like nuts, cookies and cereals that are often purchased in bulk. You can also buy these types of foods and snacks in single serving containers.

Store bread, muffins, and cookies in the freezer. This way you can take out one serving when you want it and the rest stays fresh and you won't be tempted to eat it all before it spoils.

Put the vegetables and fruits you intend to snack on at eye level in the fridge. In fact, all foods you want readily consumed from the pantry should be stored at eye level and at the front of the shelf.

Keep all food in the fridge or in the cabinets so it's out of sight. You are more likely to be tempted by food when you can see it.

Store foods you want to eat more often at the front of cabinet shelves to make it easier to grab the multigrain crackers and popcorn for a snack. You will also be less inclined to eat the sugary cereal you bought for the grandkids' visit if the high-fiber whole grain variety is the first one you see.

Schedule big food shopping trips once a week or every other week and go to the market every three to four days only when you need to replenish produce or to buy last minute ingredients. These in-between shopping trips should be quick since the produce department is near the entrance of every supermarket. Use the self-checkout and you will be in and out faster than ordering and picking up take-out.

Consider buying from at-home food delivery services like Insta-cart, Fresh Direct, and Pea Pod if food shopping in your area is less accessible or if time is a barrier to changing your food shopping habits. The positive impact on your health and decrease in health care costs may even offset any additional expense of these services.

Enlist help with the grocery runs. Check with a neighbor about alternating trips to the store, or perhaps you have a new driver in the house who would love the opportunity to get behind the wheel, even if it is only to buy eggs.

It's now time to learn about the easy changes you can make to your diet that promote healthy weight management. Get ready to learn about the benefits of eating healthy vegetable protein and the rewards of home cooking.

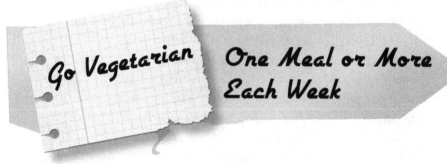

Go Vegetarian One Meal or More Each Week

An easy way to start eating healthier is to cut down on the amount of meat you eat. This can be done easily by planning to eat one vegetarian meal per week to start, like a meatless Monday. Eating vegetarian meals is easier than you might think especially if you start by just eating more beans and lentils. Beans and lentils are a low-cost, fat-free protein source and substituting a half-cup serving of beans adds fiber and essential vitamins and minerals to your diet. In fact, substituting any type of vegetable protein for animal protein, even just once a week, adds up to huge health benefits. Many tasty Mediterranean and South and Central American recipes have beans and lentils as their main ingredient. Also consider adding them to canned soups, salads, salsas, toppings, and spreads.

Another healthy low-fat vegetable protein source is tofu. Tofu is mostly used in Asian cooking, but these days more and more people are substituting it for meat in many types of recipes, including barbecue! Soy has also been shown to benefit heart health. Other research has shown soy to decrease premenopausal and menopausal symptoms in fifty percent of the women studied.

If you are not inclined to cook or are not feeling adventurous just yet, consider trying the many types of prepared products in the frozen food section made from vegetable protein, but keep an eye on the sodium content.

Vegetable fajitas, black bean and corn salads, vegetarian Bolognese sauce, and spaghetti squash primavera have become favorites of my family, which is saying a lot since my husband grew up eating only meat and potatoes.

Whole Foods vs. Convenience

It is infinitely healthier to prepare meals from scratch using whole foods than to buy ready-made ones. One of the most profound reasons for the decline in health and rise in obesity is our dependence on convenience and fast foods. The reason is that most of these foods are high in added sugar, fat, and sodium, not to mention their ever-increasing portion sizes. In addition, highly processed foods are devoid of the vitamins, minerals, and antioxidants that help us fight disease and keep our bodies at peak performance.

If you think that using convenience foods saves time, think again. A study by a nonprofit foundation found the following when researching how convenience foods are used in day-to-day life:

▶ *Convenience foods are not bought to save time, but as more elaborate meals than people normally prepare.*

▶ *Foods cooked from scratch tend to be simpler.*

> ▶ *Dinner took 30–60 minutes to get on the table no matter if it was made from scratch or a convenience food.*

The University of California, Los Angeles proved that using convenience foods doesn't put dinner on the table faster.[16] They had one group make sandwiches and salad for dinner that took thirty minutes. A second group made dinner from only convenience foods: microwaved barbecued ribs, macaroni and cheese, bagged salad, bagged dinner rolls, cookies, and ice cream for dessert That meal also took thirty minutes.

I hope this study impresses on you how preparing most of your meals and relying less on the food industry is the best way to eat properly. I caution you not to be overwhelmed anticipating the time and energy needed to shop and cook meals (especially if you've never done it). But as with doing anything new, start small and take advantage of any time you can eat a home-cooked meal instead of a fast-food or convenience meal because eating in this way will positively impact your health and your (declining) weight. Remember, this doesn't have to be an all or nothing change. Pick the one or two evenings a week when you have the time. Or, perhaps, maybe the best time to start is with a home-cooked breakfast. If that works out, move on to preparing a healthy brown-bag lunch. For those of you who have been preparing your own meals, keep reading to find tips and techniques to save time and/or improve your menu choices.

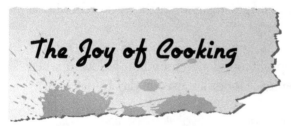

The Joy of Cooking

A while back I was developing a presentation on fast and nutritious home-cooked meals when it hit me that it takes serious time and thought to cook at home. Based on my own experience, the time it takes to shop for food, prepare brown-bag lunches for my family, and cook dinner takes an investment of time. I was also amazed how I was able to do it with the same work and family obligations as people who rely on fast and convenience foods. This led me to make several discoveries:

First was motivation. I have always been committed to providing my family with healthy, satisfying, delicious meals. Health is the main reason, but beyond that is the fact that my family actually enjoys the interaction and bonding that takes place around

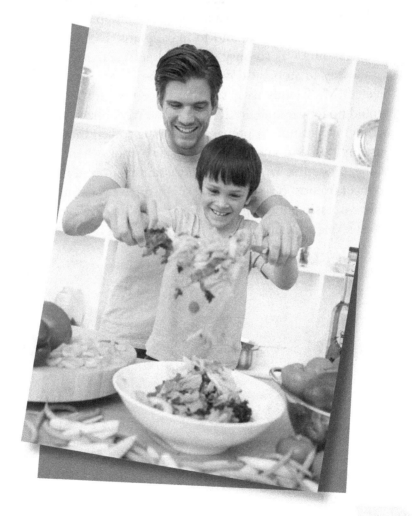

shopping, preparing, and eating food. One of my all-time favorite parenting moments came the day my ten-year-old walked into the kitchen after school and told me that something smelled really good and how she felt bad for her friends who were eating dinner at McDonald's. The truth was that I wasn't cooking anything special, but the aroma of any food cooking smells great. No convenience food can ever match it. Let's not forget that the change in your weight and your health may be the motivation you need to start cooking. I am also lucky to have an appreciative family to keep me motivated. I'm sure you may have one too.

Family dinners are also a chance to catch up on what is going on in each other's lives and to make plans. Like other modern families, ours was so busy with work and activities and dinner was a way to stop, sit down face-to-face, share—and stay connected. My friends used say that once my kids were grown, I would no longer cook in the same way. Well, I have proven them wrong. I continue to prepare most meals even though it's now just my husband and myself, but I also cook when I am eating alone. Of course without the entire family around there is time to meet friends in restaurants, usually once a week, and I am not above occasionally bringing home a salad or pizza—but the key word is occasionally.

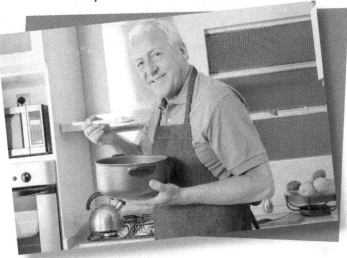

The secret as I discovered after years of cooking is that I've gotten into a routine, a rhythm, when I cook as you will also discover. For example, I often use the same ingredients. I automatically replace them when I run out, so they are always on hand.

I also prepare extra food when I have time so it's ready to eat when I am rushed or tired. Preparing extra food does not mean eating the same meal twice in a row, although that is sometimes the plan. But sometimes it means that the extra portion is intended for the next day's lunch. Another idea is to make more food than you need and freeze the rest as individual portions for lunches or dinners so there is no waste. Cooking in this way works great with soups, sauces, and stews, but you can also freeze portions of cooked chicken, fish, beef, and pork.

Another suggestion to make cooking easier is to prepare one food to use in two different ways. For example, try cooking a large batch of chicken and serve some of it one night with a baked potato and green beans. The next night cut the rest up to use in a pasta dish or for fajitas.

But keeping a well-stocked kitchen is key, so check out the appendix for a list of items that no well-stocked kitchen should be without.

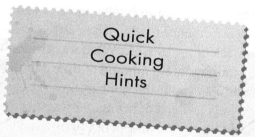

Quick
Cooking
Hints

It should come as no surprise that up to three quarters of working parents eat at least one fast food and one take-out meal per week. The reason is the scarcity of time and energy, but some home-cooked meals are just as quick, easy, and often more nutritious.

The quickest proteins to cook are fish and skinless, boneless chicken breasts which are doubly great since they are also the leanest of the animal proteins. Keep a supply of each in the freezer along with a variety of frozen vegetables just in case you run out of fresh ones. Shelf-stable canned tomato products, brown rice, quinoa, and low sodium broths are also pantry staples as are dried herbs for when fresh ones are unavailable or out of season. Citrus, mustards (especially Dijon), and vinegars are also great for imparting tasty fat-free flavor. If you like the taste of citrus in sauces, keep a few oranges or lemons in the fridge. Try to avoid canned and boxed side dishes and meal enhancers because of their high sodium content. Instead, boil quick cooking rice in low sodium broth for added flavor. Skip the Hamburger Helper and Knorr Pasta Sides and cook your protein in whole foods, such as canned tomatoes, and vegetables (fresh, frozen, or canned), seasoned with fresh or dried herbs.

Several years ago, Margaret Beck, archaeologist, and anthropologist, as a postdoctoral scholar at UCLA's Center on Every Day Lives of Families, studied how long it took to prepare meals. She found that almost all home-cooked meals included packaged convenience foods such as jarred pasta sauce, frozen vegetables, stir-fry mixes, etc. What was even more interesting is that she found that the amount of time it took to get the meal on the table was about the same as those cooked totally from scratch. What's more, it didn't matter whether 20 or 50 percent of the meal was from convenience items. The bottom line was that using convenience foods saved only ten minutes of prep time. It seems that convenience foods don't save time so much as allow for the preparation of more elaborate meals.

When you are trying a new recipe, look for dishes with five ingredients or less or those with few cooking steps. If a more involved recipe catches your eye, save it for a weekend, that's what I do. Remember that making a recipe for the first time is more time consuming than it will be after you've made it once or twice.

Experiment in the kitchen. Try baking chicken instead of frying it. It's not only healthier, but you just may enjoy it more that way. When looking for recipe ideas, try entering the names of the ingredients you have on hand into a Google search or one of many recipe sites like www.tasteofhome.com and www.cookstr. com. You will be amazed to find recipes that fit the bill. Most of us tend to stick to eating familiar foods always prepared in much the same way. We are creatures of habit. However, since you're looking to control portion size, maybe shaking up the taste buds is just the ticket. This way you will have a greater variety of tastes in your home-cooked meals than in your favorite already-prepared food—where the taste never varies. If you are not adventurous with food, no problem, just stay with what you like. The food prep of a familiar recipe is faster, and your familiarity with it allows for making variations, like substituting broth for some of the fat or including more or different vegetables. Your goal is not only to prepare much of the food yourself, but also to make it tasty and satisfying.

So, to get started get out your pen and paper or open your note-taking app of choice, and make a shopping list, and don't forget to make sure you have the correct utensils and gadgets you might need to make preparing your food as effortless as possible.

Speeding Up Food Prep

► *Start with what takes the longest to cook. Brown rice needs to simmer for forty minutes, but the fish bakes in twelve, so start the rice first.*

► *Do the peeling and chopping first. When I make my family's favorite chicken primavera over pasta, I start by chopping the peppers, mushrooms, tomato and broccoli on one cutting board and the chicken on a separate cutting board before I even take a pot out of the cabinet.*

► *Keep knives sharp. Dull knives cause accidents.*

► *Get family members to help. An extra pair of hands for chopping or stirring is a real time saver, even if it is just for a couple of minutes.*

► *Preheat the oven. Turn It on to heat up as soon as you walk in the door.*

► *Buy fresh or frozen pre-sliced or chopped ingredients. You can even find chopped onions and herbs In the freezer section of your supermarket to make meals more flavorful.*

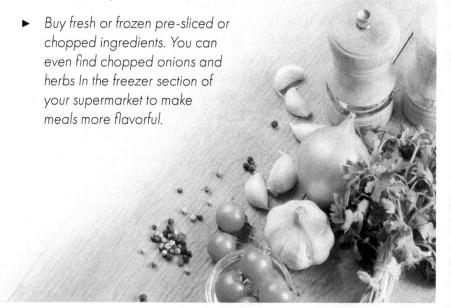

- Stock up on extra sets of measuring cups and spoons as well as bowls, cutting boards, cooking utensils, and knives so you don't have to stop and wash between uses.

- Assemble all ingredients in one area. before you start cooking. This way you're not running around the kitchen pulling things out of draws and the fridge.

- Stock up on low-sodium canned goods, including tomato products and broths.

- Use what's on hand or learn to substitute. If you don't have leeks or shallots, use an onion.

- Marinate in zip-seal bags, that way there is no dish to wash.

- Buy thin cuts of chicken and meat because they cook faster.

- Buy pre-cooked chicken breasts like Perdue Short Cuts which are healthier and more versatile than rotisserie and deli chicken selections.

- Invest in a food processor and don't forget the mini which makes quick work of chopping everything from herbs to vegetables to nuts.

- Consider an indoor electric grill. This amazing appliance gets a flavorful dinner on the table in minutes. All you need is a little bottled dressing, marinade, rub or glaze and chicken, or fish. It is also works great for turkey, salmon, and beef burgers. If you're cooking for one, they also come in small sizes.

▶ *Stock up on quick-cooking side dishes. Quick-cooking rice, microwaved "baked" potatoes, fresh veggies or frozen vegetables for steaming or sauteing, and pre-made salads all work when you don't have time to fuss.*

▶ *Keep a supply of frozen burgers, canned tuna, and low-sodium canned soups, (or frozen homemade) and you'll always be able to make a quick meal of soup and a sandwich.*

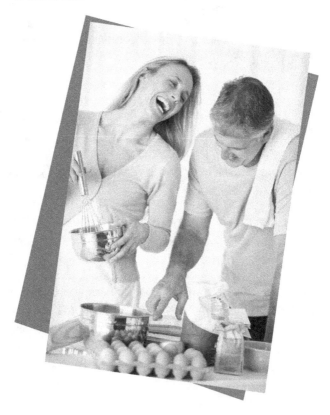

In addition, to make home cooking even easier, don't be bashful about asking others in your household who are benefitting from your cooking to help you get meals on the table or to do the dishes. Or maybe you need someone to stop on their way home to pick up a few groceries. Tonight I am going to serve some leftover meatloaf I have stored in the freezer with a side of spaghetti squash and vegetables I made last night. The only thing I need to prepare is a salad. What are you having for dinner?

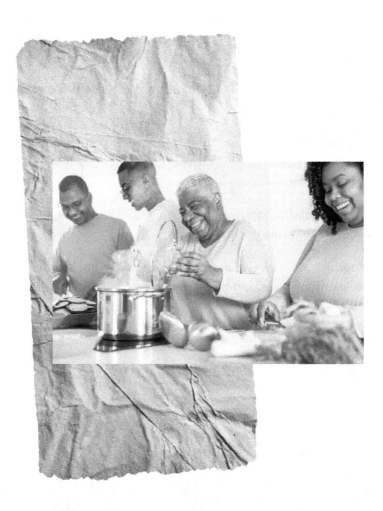

Your Goals for This Week:

1. Practice reading food labels

2. Devise a convenient and easy method for keeping and adding to your shopping list for planning meals or to keep track of staple items you've run out of

3. Decide which days are best to food shop and which are best to cook

4. Purchase or organize multiple sizes of food storage containers, cooking utensils, and kitchen gadgets to help make cooking as effortless as possible

5. Declutter and organize kitchen cabinets to make often-used foods more easily accessible

5. Stock up on foods and ingredients that will increase your likelihood of preparing meals at home

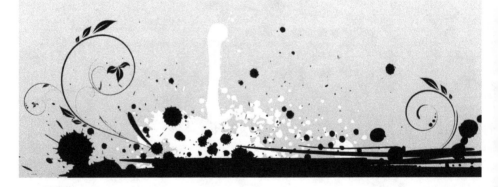

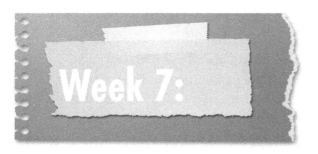

Stay on Track When Eating Out

Since you have been working on preparing meals at home for the past week, this means you have also navigated through a weekend. The reason I am mentioning this is because for many of us, weekend meals mean dining out or eating take-out which, if we're not careful, can ruin a weight loss plan. I often hear from people that even though they watch their food intake all week, they are apt to undo any progress by making poor food choices on weekends. This behavior plays a big part in yo-yo cycling—when weight keeps going up and down. The best way to stop this cycle is to apply your newly acquired eating habits to what you eat when you eat out and what you order when you order in. Once you take charge of your eating habits when mastering these types of eating, you will be able to continue your weight loss efforts. In fact, you'll be able to eat an occasional restaurant meal out or enjoy a weeklong vacation and maintain your healthy eating habits. Over the years, I have helped many people on this program celebrate not only losing (and continuing to lose) weight, but also those who maintained that weight loss. What they all had in common was learning how to order or choose food wisely from a menu, at a buffet table, or from a tray at a cocktail party. Oh, and making wise food choices also requires specific techniques for holiday eating, too.

Celebrating Doesn't Make Us Fat

I once saw a list of weight-loss recommendations that advised people who were watching their weight not to participate in social occasions. I was appalled! To think that in order to reach a health goal meant forgoing meals with family and friends and to not celebrate special occasions is just too much for any of us to tolerate. It's exactly this type of draconian rule that makes people not want to diet. Dieting, by its very nature, can be isolating, so I believe that it's best to learn behaviors that support health goals no matter what day (or holiday) it happens to be. After all, life is filled with many challenging situations and in order to succeed in your weight-loss quest, you need to learn how to conquer them by doing them. As they say, "practice makes perfect." I will now show you what you need to know in order to use every restaurant meal or party situation as a learning experience. You may not get it all right at the start, or even every time, but the success of this program relies on trial and correction, not trial and error.

I happen to be writing this chapter on my laptop at a New York airport waiting for a flight to California. That is quite a long trip to make without eating, but I am actually relieved that the airlines stopped serving meals on domestic flights because it makes it acceptable for passengers to bring their own healthier food choices on board. I pack my lunch and a snack in my carry-on. However, on this trip I noticed there were more prepared food choices available in the terminal. (Yes, I know—It's an occupational hazard, I guess!) Even though the quality of airport food has improved—at least at some airports—it's not a good idea to rely on always being able to find a healthy, well-balanced meal there. The bottom line is that if you find yourself in need of having to buy prepared food when traveling, it is now possible.

Eating Healthy When Dining Out

It doesn't matter if you're eating fast food, fast casual, or dining in a fine restaurant, eating out can potentially lead to poor meal choices. For example, how do you know the fat, sugar, or sodium content of foods unless you either prepared them yourself or they come with a food label? Restaurant portions are also notorious for being on the large side which encourages eating more than we normally would because the more food on our plate, the better the chance we will eat it—all.

But the Federal Food and Drug Administration (FDA) has stepped up to the plate, so to speak, and now require food establishments with more than 20 locations to post nutrition labels for their menu items. Don't get too excited as this is not always an accurate account as a report in the *Journal of the American Dietetic Association* found out. They documented the number of calories in some foods were higher than indicated, sometimes by as much as 18 percent.[17] What's more, the food items in that study were selected because they had fewer than 500 calories. Not only were these among the lowest calorie items on the menu, but they were also more than likely have been the items specifically chosen by customers watching their calories. Also be aware that the US FDA allows up to 20 percent error in calorie reporting. This means that you always need to be vigilant because even the nutrition labels in restaurants are often misleading.

Nevertheless, one of the best tools for eating healthy out is the nutrition label. Consulting this label before you order helps you make the best food choices. But again, beware! Any purchased meal could contain hidden calories and this is in addition to any inaccurately reported calories as well as side dishes not even being included in the final tally of nutrition facts. Not to worry. I am here to give you a map for successfully navigating the minefield of eating out without sabotaging your weight-loss efforts.

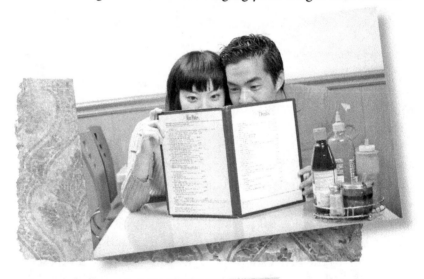

Mapping Your Dining-Out Strategy

The behaviors supportive of weight loss begin before you leave home for the restaurant, which means that on the days you plan to eat out, you should never skip a meal or snack, thinking you will save calories. This happens when you automatically think of restaurant eating as overeating when in truth it's skipping a meal or snack that sets you up to be overly hungry and in less control when it comes to ordering and eating mindfully. Being overly hungry also makes you less likely to tap into or follow hunger/fullness cues, or to follow portion control, eat slowly, or practice other healthy eating habits. Skipping a meal or snack thinking it will save calories actually encourages eating more. Since restaurant food is often higher in calories than the equivalent food prepared at home, eating out is not the best time to clean your plate. Again, extreme hunger always leads to poor food choices and eating too quickly makes it impossible for the brain to signal when you are full.

The absolute best thing to do when eating out is to eat slowly enough to follow hunger/fullness cues so you know when you are satisfied. Do this and you make it possible to resist the temptation to clean your plate. What you don't eat you can take home to enjoy again, maybe as lunch the next day.

Another technique you can use to avoid overeating when confronted with a large restaurant portion is to divide the meal in half as soon as it put in front of you—before you even take the first bite. That dividing line on your plate marks the point where you should ask yourself, "Am I still hungry?" I have a friend who asks the server to put half of his meal in a take-out container before it is even brought to the table. Another thing you can do to reduce the temptation to continue eating once you are full is to position your utensils across the plate with the handles touching the leftover food. This makes it less likely you'll pick them up again to keep eating.

Size Does Matter

Restaurants want you to feel you are getting good value for your money which translates to portions large enough for two meals. We have gotten so used to seeing these large portions that we now think of them as standard-size meals when the truth is these large meals often contain a full day's worth of calories.

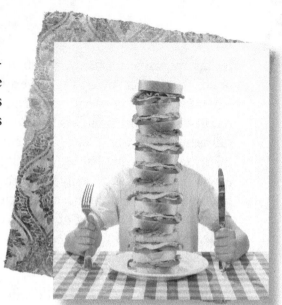

Weight as a Socially Transmitted Disease

Don't laugh, it's true. Social norms do influence what and how much we eat. When those around us choose high-calorie foods, it significantly increases our chances of doing the same. Social norms also influence how much we eat. Knowing this will help you resist temptation when you eat with people—who eat large high-calorie meals and snacks. You'll know to not let the actions of others negatively influence or derail your food decisions, weight loss, and health.

On the other hand, following social norms is not always a bad thing, especially when you share meals or belong to a group or community who eat healthy. Just as you may be influenced to make poor choices you can also be influenced to eat healthier when around people who do exactly that. Like it or not, our food decisions are influenced by those we identify with and this behavior even carries over to the food choices we make when eating alone.

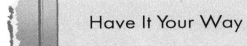

Have It Your Way

You do not need to sacrifice taste to avoid overeating. With a little detective work and some proactive ordering, you can avoid many overeating food traps. Here's how:

Avoid eating appetizers before the main course. Appetizers often contain more calories than an entire meal. If you see something you can't resist, share it, or order it as your main course. Appetizers are smaller plate options and are often interesting flavor combinations or food pairings that are very satisfying. They are often a sufficient amount of food especially when paired with a salad or a hearty soup.

Order salad as an appetizer. Studies show that starting a meal with a low-fat (not Caesar) salad decreases the overall number of calories consumed. It is also a great way to get in another daily serving of veggies. Ask that your salad to be served immediately so you won't be tempted to dive into the breadbasket. Remember to ask for the dressing, preferably a vinaigrette or any other that is low in fat, to be served on the side.

Avoid high-calorie salad add-ons. For example, croutons, Asian noodles, and fried toppings are not an option because they add extra calories and fat. The rule Is that the only crunchy ingredients in a salad should be

from plants. Instead consider healthy additions such as nuts, fruit, and beans. If a regular dressing is your only choice, or there is a dressing you just can't resist, have it served on the side and dip your fork in the dressing before using it to pick up a bite of salad. This ensures that you will taste the dressing with each bite without needlessly saturating the salad greens. You will be surprised at how flavorful a salad can be even without using a lot of dressing. If you're not in the mood for a salad or not really a salad person, then an alternative smart choice is to order a broth-based soup.

Steer clear of the breadbasket. If you truly cannot resist, eat only one slice or one small roll and skip the butter or margarine. Instead ask for some olive oil for dipping (same number of calories, but heart-healthy). If you find you can't resist a second slice, ask the wait staff to remove the rest.

Order first. Do this and you won't be tempted by what everyone else chooses.

Choose from the light menu if one is available. Light entrées are carefully constructed with the health conscious in mind and designed not to be bland and boring. Sometimes it is helpful to know what to order even before you enter the restaurant. This gives you the benefit of decreasing the amount of time spent perusing the delicious sounding, though less healthful, menu choices. You'll find menus posted on the restaurant's website. Knowing what you'll order ahead of time has the added benefit of helping you look forward to that meal and increasing the chances that if you've decided on baked chicken that your eye will automatically find that selection jump off the page when you actually read the menu in person. This strategy decreases your chances of being distracted by the fried chicken or cheeseburger.

Ask Questions and don't be afraid to make special requests. Quiz your waiter about the cooking method. Is butter or oil added? Is there cream or butter in the sauce? Can you substitute steamed vegetables or a salad for French fries? Don't be afraid to ask that food be broiled or grilled instead of the cooking method listed. Request that oil, salt, or cream not be added and that sauces and dressings be served on the side. Instead of a starch consider an extra side of vegetables.

Most restaurants will accommodate these types of requests. If they cannot, well, nothing ventured, nothing gained, but always ask. You should be able to get your meal the way you want it and the restaurant is there to serve you.

Always avoid anything described as crispy, crunchy, cheesy, or creamy. Carefully reading menu descriptions as to how each dish is prepared helps you make healthier choices. Safe bets include dishes described as baked, roasted, grilled, broiled, poached, blackened, boiled, steamed, broth, marinara, filet, kebab, or top sirloin. Stay away from the fat traps like au gratin, en croute, croquette, pan-fried, crispy, breaded, creamed, stewed, buttered, prime beef, pot pie, casserole, beurre blanc, and alfredo.

Drink water. If you're not a fan of plain water, jazz it up by requesting slices of lemon or order a bottle of sparkling water instead. A 5-ounce glass of red wine is a wise chosen splurge, but the 400-calorie margarita is counterproductive. Avoid sugared soft drinks and alcoholic cocktails which have a surprisingly large number of calories, as the above-mentioned margarita makes clear.

Get creative with dessert. Instead of a traditional high-calorie dessert, order a skim milk cappuccino or fresh berries (hold the cream), nonfat yogurt, or sorbet. A baked apple or almond biscotti are also smart choices. For those times when you cannot resist a high-calorie dessert, share it with the table or your dining companion. Often, just a bite or two of something sweet is all you need for a satisfying finish to a great meal.

By practicing these eating behaviors you'll come to regard dining out as a refreshing change and not something to fear as a threat to your weight loss efforts.

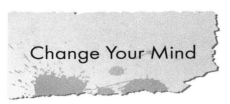

Change Your Mind

It's important that you remember that dining out should be a joyful experience centered around meeting and spending time with friends or family. Do not let anxiety over food choices limit you from getting out. Dining out is also an opportunity to eat leisurely and be served meals you don't have to shop for or prepare (or do the dishes afterwards). It is a meal (or an event or a celebration) in pleasant surroundings and a rare opportunity to feel cared for and literally waited on. So focus on these positive aspects of eating out, and not on the food you are ordering and eating. Changing your perspective also helps make it easier to choose healthier menu items or to eat smaller portions.

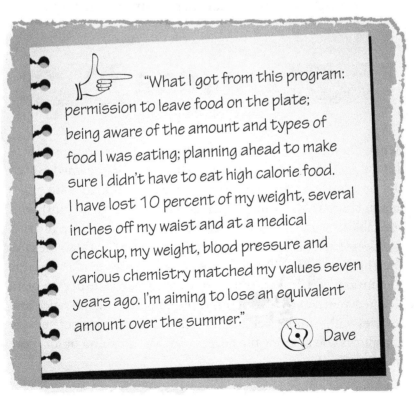

"What I got from this program: permission to leave food on the plate; being aware of the amount and types of food I was eating; planning ahead to make sure I didn't have to eat high calorie food. I have lost 10 percent of my weight, several inches off my waist and at a medical checkup, my weight, blood pressure and various chemistry matched my values seven years ago. I'm aiming to lose an equivalent amount over the summer."

Dave

Italian

Better choices include minestrone, bean soup, seafood salad, marinated calamari, steamed mussels, any pasta with tomato sauce, marinara sauce, clam sauce, puttanesca, or primavera sauce, veal, or chicken marsala, cacciatore or piccata, any baked or broiled fish, or pizza with vegetable topping. Avoid cream sauces, cheese as a main ingredient, pancetta, and sausage.

CHINESE

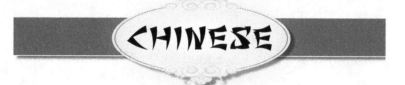

Better choices are wonton soup, hot and sour soup, steamed dumplings, steamed vegetables, stir-fried or steamed sliced chicken, beef, or seafood with vegetables, lo mein with vegetables, chicken or shrimp, steamed rice, bean curd (tofu) with vegetables, or moo shu chicken or shrimp. Steer clear of fried and deep-fried dishes like fried rice and egg rolls. Watch the rice. Even brown rice is 240 calories per cup. Portions tend to be large so consider sharing an entrée and get an extra order of plain steamed vegetables. Mixing together an entrée full of sauce and calories with more vegetables decreases the calories per serving and allows you to enjoy the flavors with a companion or for more than one meal.

JAPANESE

Miso soup, clear soup, braised or grilled beef, chicken or fish, chicken teriyaki, stir-fried, steamed, or pickled vegetables, tofu dishes, and steamed rice may be good picks. Keep in mind sushi varies from thirty to seventy calories per piece. A five-piece California roll contains 140 calories.

MEXICAN

Choose gazpacho, black bean soup, salsa, enchiladas, burritos, soft tacos with chicken, seafood, or vegetables, or chicken fajitas. High-fat proteins like beef, pork, and cheese may be obvious poor choices. But consider how many calories the tacos, tortillas, guacamole, and rice can add to even a well-designed meal.

Steakhouse

Better selections include French onion soup without cheese, Manhattan clam chowder, shrimp cocktail, London broil, filet mignon, plain baked potato, steamed vegetables, broiled or baked seafood, or broiled or baked breast of chicken. Prime rib, rib-eye, and porterhouse steaks will give you a whole day's worth of fat on that one plate. You could try limiting your portion to six ounces or you could choose the filet mignon or the grilled tuna steak instead. Be mindful of the butter on the baked potato (order it without and add a little on your own), the cream in the spinach (better you order it sautéed), and the calories and fat in the blue cheese dressing that will turn the attempt to reduce calorie intake by ordering the salad first into a fat fest. Instead opt for a vinaigrette dressing to be served on the side.

Wishing You Happy and Healthy Holidays

When I present this program to a live audience, I make sure to include the following section just prior to a major holiday. If you're not reading this near a holiday, feel free to skim through it and mark the pages that you think most apply to you. That way you can easily find this section when you truly need it.

I encourage people to go easy on themselves during the holidays by eating mindfully and practicing new eating habits, but to not sacrifice the celebration or the company of family and friends, or in any way take away from the enjoyment that holidays bring to our lives. My advice is to set a realistic holiday goal to not regain any lost weight. I remember one year when just before Thanksgiving we offered massage gift certificates to any

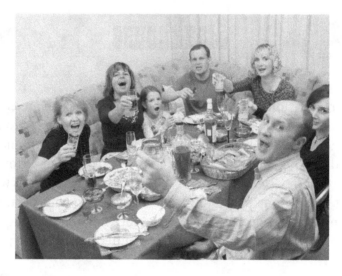

audience participant who weighed in after New Year's at their pre-Thanksgiving weight. Not only did more than half the group win that free massage, but the majority also maintained their weight loss with some losing even more weight. Wow! Now it's your turn. Would a free massage be enough to help you continue your weight loss efforts despite a birthday or family feast? Then I suggest you stay motivated and keep your goals realistic, doable, and measurable and feel free to use a reward system to keep your eye on the prize, so to speak.

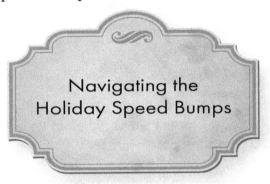

Navigating the Holiday Speed Bumps

If you make a list of all the holidays both religious and secular, including everything from Super Bowl Sunday to St. Patrick's Day and add in birthdays, anniversaries, weddings, bar mitzvahs, and christenings, you will find 2.4 chances to feast every month. Think about how every one of these occasions can affect your food choices (and do away with the myth that the weight-gaining holidays are only in December). The list of challenges is endless: hors d'oeuvres, buffets, several invitations in one weekend, alcohol, tempting desserts, feeling left out or different, guests in your home, being a guest, less time, more shopping, more cooking, more wrapping, and more baking.

Just as you make a choice when you come to any fork in the road, your road to healthy eating also comes with having to make choices as to which path (food) to choose. Make the choices that will lead you to a successful end. All you need to do is plan ahead to make it easier to choose the right path and avoid any speed bumps and potholes that threaten to slow your progress. Here are some suggestions:

Mark all special events on a calendar. This helps with time management and also alerts you to anticipate making mindful food choices. Whether looking up a menu online ahead of time or packing an extra snack to hold off your hunger during an ordinary workday.

Snack before you leave home or keep healthy snacks handy in your office or car to eat before the event. A snack to control hunger decreases the chance of being tempted to taste anything and everything that comes your way. Good snack choices include an apple, Greek or regular yogurt, 3 cups air-popped popcorn, 1-ounce of pretzels, 8 almonds, or a low-fat granola bar.

Do not skip meals in preparation for a holiday meal or celebration. Attending a party hungry will lead to making poor food choices and Increases your chances of overeating.

Balance eating a heavier high-calorie restaurant or celebratory meal with lighter, lower-fat foods for the remainder of the day. Try turkey on whole wheat with lettuce and tomato for lunch if you expect to attend a dinner party or choose grilled chicken over low-fat salad for dinner if you've eaten an elaborate lunch.

Hors d'oeuvres and appetizers present the perfect opportunity for mindless eating, so limit your choices and stick to those that are not laden with fat, sugar, and lots of calories. Resolve ahead of time the amount you will eat and limit your choices to those made with vegetables, fruit, chicken, or fish—and none that have been fried or drowned in cream or cheese sauces. Other sensible choices are those that contain high-fiber grains in small portions. Also hold onto your dirty napkin or plate as a reminder that you have already eaten.

Socialize and circulate to keep your distance from the food and minimize temptation. Avoid being near the kitchen door at all costs. Sitting or standing on either side of that door will give you a bird's-eye view of every hors d'oeuvre and put you first in line to eat them.

Brighten up holiday tables with colorful, healthy fresh produce. Serve veggies with assorted low-fat dips. Serve fresh fruit salad or cooked compotes instead of or in addition to cakes and pies.

Think of a cookie or two as a complete dessert. Cookies offer variety in small bites and fewer calories.

Bring a low-fat appetizer or fruit dessert to a gathering to assure you have at least one healthy choice. (If you are like me, I can't walk into someone's home empty-handed, and this suggestion kills two birds with one stone.)

You don't have to eat (or taste) everything in order to enjoy yourself. When you are confronted with a wide variety of food, make conscious choices as to which ones you will eat. It also doesn't hurt to <u>consciously remind</u> yourself that you don't have to eat everything in order to have a good time.

Eat only your favorite foods or those that are holiday specific. Do not waste your calories on foods you can eat any time of the year. For instance, at Thanksgiving dinner, consider that mashed potatoes are on the menu all year long, but sweet potato pie and turkey stuffing are special to the holiday. This makes it easy to skip foods like mashed potatoes and concentrate on eating a small portion of your favorite foods that celebrate the season or are holiday specific.

Attend to hunger and fullness cues. Start with small portions, eat slowly, and savor every bite. Holiday meals include a lot of chatting, so use this time to give your stomach the twenty minutes It needs to talk to your brain. Try not to get distracted by the other diners. Stay focused, and if you listen to your body, it will tell you when it is satisfied. Stop eating before you feel full. If you cannot leave the table, place your napkin in or over your plate so you aren't tempted to keep eating.

Make a list of your health goals and chosen behavior changes and review it often during the days of holiday eating. Be diligent about keeping up your food journal. Use non-food rewards for your successes.

Exercise. Schedule exercise time as you would any appointment. Exercise is often the first thing we forgo when we get busy. Don't forget that exercise not only burns those extra holiday calories, but it also helps with the added stress the holidays may bring.

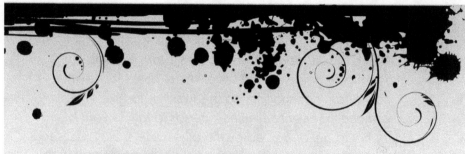

Your Goals for This Week, or Weekend, Upcoming Event, Holiday, or Vacation:

1. Make a list of the behavior changes that will help influence how you prepare for and navigate restaurant meals and events that serve food. If there are too many to change at once, start small and change one or two at a time.

2. Use the behavior chain technique to identify the actions necessary to affect a positive outcome

3. Practice mindful eating at all holiday events, no matter what the surroundings

4. Maintain your food logs

5. Stick to your exercise regimen as closely as possible

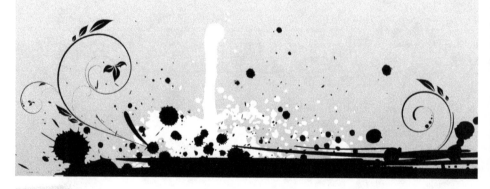

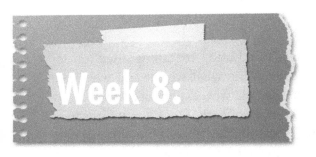

Week 8:

Social Sand Traps

The social sand traps I am referring to are the food traps placed in our way by the well-meaning people in our lives who know us well enough to say:

"Just have a taste."

"The rest of the office is going out to lunch and you're going to the gym?"

"What! You don't like your mother's soup?"

"Come on, one bite won't hurt you."

"You are going for a walk? What about me?"

Eating Underminers

Support from others may increase weight loss success and may be critical in the weight maintenance phase of weight loss, however, many of us live in an environment where the value and efforts we have placed on eating right and exercising may not be shared with most of the people close to us.[18] These family members, friends, and significant others apply the most social pressure in eating situations. Their comments and encouragements to eat only serves to increase our dissatisfaction with our weight and the focus placed on it in addition to calling attention to any decisions we make concerning what we eat and when we eat it. Research shows that people who experience this type of eating-undermining eat more frequently. Once you understand that making small changes to your diet make a big difference in your overall calorie intake, then it stands to reason that you need strategies to cope with eating underminers who can encourage you to consume an extra 100–200 calories to (often) more than several hundred calories when you're around them. An eating underminer can keep your weight loss efforts stuck in neutral or, even worse, in reverse.

Rehearsing Planned Responses to Stay on Track

Let's face it, some of us are more sensitive to undermining comments and behaviors while others are merely surrounded by more people who negatively influence behavior choices. No matter which camp you're in, rehearsing a planned response to dealing with these underminers is key to staying on track.

But before we begin, it's important that you identify the specific situation, environment, or person that poses the greatest challenge. You may find it helpful to review the list of triggers you listed in the behavior chain exercise (see Chapter 5). Think about what makes you lose your focus. Is it what someone says, how they say it, or the response you give that impacts your behavior? Keep in mind that a response can be verbal, an action, or a feeling. In all of these cases, the best response is the one that is the most succinct if it is to be successful. The point is to stop the triggered behavior by avoiding all further discussion or explanation. This is the result you need in order to stay on track and maintain your weight loss focus.

Remember, too, that the people who sabotage your health efforts often have good intentions and mean you no harm, so staying polite and gracious is in everyone's best interest. Say something positive to acknowledge their gesture and offer an alternative to avoid another comment (or to dissuade a pusher).

One woman who sought my help with weight loss had the challenge of working in an office where the staff brought in baked goods daily and left them on the counter in the break room. She was very overweight and expressed to me feeling self-conscious around her coworkers. She had even overheard them comment to one another about her weight. This situation made her feel if she took a cookie they would make negative comments, if she didn't, it would call attention to her weight. Also, the healthy behavior she was working on was to eat a piece of fruit as her snack to improve her nutrient intake and control calories. The constant visible supply of cookies, brownies, and candy was an obstacle for her. Her solution of planned response was this: When a coworker would say "Jane, have some cookies." She would reply "Thanks, I'm not hungry right now but I will take it with me for later." She would put the cookie on a napkin, carry it to her desk, and throw it in the trash.

My Soup Challenge

I have found myself in a challenging situation every holiday with my family. My mother is a wonderful cook and sets out food for thirty when she is expecting twelve. I have, in the past, found that by the middle of the main course, I have eaten past the point of satiety and because everything tastes so good and because there is a lot of encouragement from my relatives to keep eating, that I am an uncomfortable ten on the hunger/fullness scale.

One holiday I decided that it was time to change my behavior. I thought through what foods I could eliminate or limit with the goal of comfortably enjoying the meal and the rest of the evening that followed. I chose to skip the soup course and asked my mother to put some in a container for me to take home to enjoy for lunch the following day. That first holiday, and come to think of it the second as well, with spoons in hand, someone at the table yelled out "Wait, Amy doesn't have any soup. Why aren't you eating soup? What's the matter with you? What, you don't like your mother's soup?" So at first, I launched into a whole explanation of why I was not having soup. This actually led to not

only listening to the same uncomfortable verbal assaults every holiday, but some well-meaning relatives began to monitor everything I put on my plate. But, as I explained above, a simply worded phrase changed everything.

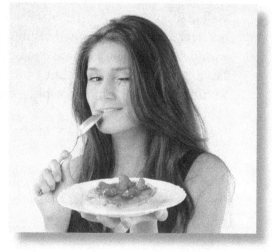

Now, every year when the same questions start when the soup is served I say, "Thanks for thinking of me, but I am passing on the soup for now." As an aside, my husband or my daughter have taken to asking me if I want a taste of theirs to make me feel included and that makes me feel respected and cared for.

Some Planned Responses

If you are not hungry when others invite you to eat, simply say, "Thanks for asking, I'll have some tea and keep you company."

If you are offered a snack, say, "Thanks I am going to pass for now."

Or "Thank you, I'll have some a little later."

If you are offered a home-baked treat, say, "It looks and smells great. Can I have the recipe?" Or "Can I take some home?"

A polite reply to your hostess is to say, "Thanks, I'm full. I am going to wait for dessert for now."

If you are invited to join groups of friends or coworkers for lunches too often for comfort, think about accepting an invitation once a week for your social life or your team-building efforts. Then go online and review the menu for the best food choices. Or plan time on those days before or after work to do aerobic exercise.

Most important is that you think through your challenge and plan a kind and thoughtful response that also includes an alternative behavior (for you) completing a strategy to improve the outcome.

Getting Physical

The Energy Gap

The energy gap has to do with the not so slight imbalances between calorie consumption and calorie burn that lead to weight gain. Most of us know it as eating more calories than we burn. The energy gap is especially common during vacations and holidays when eating extra calories is more frequent and for more days in a row than the occasional splurge. No matter when you overindulge, the only way not to gain weight is to increase the frequency and duration of physical activity to burn off extra calories.

In fact, exercise is the common denominator shared by all successful long-term weight maintainers as evidenced by The National Weight Loss Registry which cites exercise as the integral factor of members who have maintained their weight loss for one plus years.

As we learned in the previous chapter, exercise is also a great stress reducer during an event and especially during the holidays.

The best way to evaluate how well your exercise routine is impacting your weight loss is to make sure to significantly challenge yourself during your workouts. If your workouts are not yielding results, then it's time to adjust their frequency, duration, and intensity.

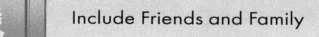

Include Friends and Family

One important and overlooked aspect to exercising is its social component, which affects exercise in much in the same way as it does eating. This is because of the real ability of others to help us maintain healthy behaviors. This is well documented in people who exercise regularly and how they benefit immensely from the support of their workout buddies and the encouragement of partners who may or may not also be workout buddies.

One Thanksgiving I invited my daughter to join me on a walk around the neighborhood before the rest of the family arrived. I told her it was because I wanted time to visit with her alone, but it was really because I needed physical activity to relieve my back pain. We enjoyed our walk so much that we have made it a Thanksgiving tradition. So never underestimate the positive influence others have over your exercise habits—the ones who actually exercise with you and the ones who encourage you to keep at it.

I want you to be aware that exercise also harbors underminers. Yes, these people will sabotage the efforts of others and they seem to be as plentiful as eating underminers. Just as you would with eating underminers, compose a statement that clearly states your desire not to mess with your exercise schedule. This will remove any pressure being put on you to concede to others wishes and instead will increase your conviction.

One year when my daughter and I were preparing to leave the house for our Thanksgiving walk, my husband questioned why I was leaving when I had dinner to prepare. I answered by saying that I planned to be back in thirty minutes and could he please turn the oven on in fifteen so I could start cooking the turkey as soon as I got home. It worked beautifully. Short and friendly and true with no for further comment needed.

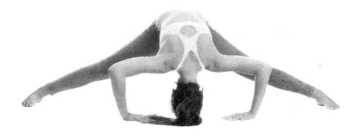

Go the Extra Mile

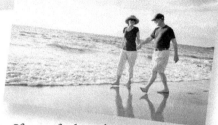

I guarantee that you will be delightfully surprised at the difference increasing your walking or biking time to ten minutes from five or doing aerobics five times a week instead of four makes. If you feel you've reached the limit of your current exercise routine, then add a new one. (Notice that I said "add" not replace.) Increasing your physical activity by adding a new sport or activity may even provide you with an opportunity to include friends and family.

I wanted to take tennis lessons, but since the only time I had was the time my husband and I had set aside to spend together, we decided to both take lessons. This led to us spending a few hours together each week while getting healthy at the same time. Keep in mind that tennis lessons were *in addition* to my regular exercise regimen. My mother even asked to join us when she visited. My husband and I both got more physical activity, and I got to spend more time with my mom, too. My daughter began to take lessons so I also got to practice with her. These days I play an occasional Sunday morning set with a friend which combines exercising with catching up. Choose an activity you love and you'll find that there is no downside.

If you don't know where to start, check out what your local community center, public school adult education sessions, or your local library has to offer. And don't forget the internet where you can find both individual instruction and group fitness classes on streaming service providers and platforms like Zoom. This added convenience makes it possible to exercise on your own schedule or from a local studio or any other spot on the globe without ever leaving home. For those with a bigger budget, Mirror, NordicTrack iFit, and Peloton offer a diverse selection of classes, fitness levels, and exercise choices.

Always remember that the point is also to increase your exercise goals as you get leaner and stronger. And adding a new activity prevents boredom and provides a challenge to your muscles which in turn burns additional calories.

Be adventurous. Revisit any barriers that kept you from trying new things in the past. If you find physical exercise embarrassing, get a DVD or bring up a routine on YouTube or Fit TV and dance or exercise at home. Once you gain confidence, you'll feel better about joining a class or a gym. Chances are you'll make new friends who were probably just as apprehensive as you. If lack of time keeps you from exercising, then choose a weekend activity. Don't forget about walking or biking to work if that's an option. Try turning exercise time into family time with hiking, yoga, rock-climbing, basketball, kayaking, or any other activity the family will enjoy doing together.

For some of you, weight might also cause discomfort to hips, knees, feet, and the respiratory system. But don't let that

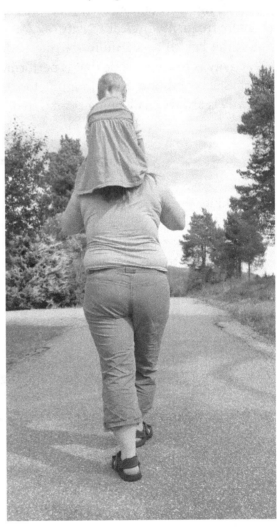

stop you. Some people begin by doing exercises while sitting on a chair. Others, who are more able, start by taking short walks. Consider swimming at the local pool as swimming has the added benefit of taking pressure off the joints.

Get moving and you'll be pleasantly surprised that in as little as two months, you can lose enough weight to make movement easier. I've seen it happen many times. It's amazing how the simple act of moving increases stamina and melts away pounds. The resulting new comfort level promotes longer, more intense, and more frequent physical activity.

The key to successfully starting and maintaining a planned activity is to choose one that is performed easily in your *current* physical condition. Keep in mind, too, that starting any new activity is always challenging at first, so don't get discouraged.

Choosing an Activity

Walking, cycling, and swimming allow you to move at your own pace. However, they tend to be solitary activities unless you join a club or ask someone to join you. For a more social exercising experience, there's always aerobics, tai chi, or yoga classes. Just remember, choose an activity you enjoy so it's a positive experience and will allow you to stay motivated.

I know it can be tough if you're not used to exercising in the company of others, but don't let it stop you. There is no reason to ever feel embarrassed. For one, you have no way of knowing at what level of experience or conditioning the others in the class began and how far they have progressed. Yes, you may be larger than they are now, but chances are they are thinking encouraging thoughts like "good for him" and "you go, girl." You just may be in for a few surprises if you get out there and exercise. I'm laying odds that you'll meet others who have experienced what you are now feeling. Remember never to underestimate the social power of exercise.

I once had the pleasure of counseling a woman who was very deconditioned due to multiple medical problems. Even though exercise was essential for her health, her limited resources and many physical barriers made it difficult to come up with a plan. One thing she did not lack was a positive attitude and this made all the difference. Through my recommendation, she got a free membership to the local YMCA which had a fitness center and a pool. Even though she didn't know how to swim, I still suggested she get into the water and hold on to the side and kick her legs. I really admired her as she was able to put aside her embarrassment and found she enjoyed being in that pool so much that she went every day. Her presence also inspired other older adults to follow her example and before long she had company. One of the instructors offered her swimming lessons, and the personal trainer developed an exercise routine geared to strength training for her to do in the gym. This success story began with finding the courage to try something new (and I hear these stories all the time). If you're in this position, ask yourself "Is losing weight worth some minor discomfort?" Your only answer should be a resounding "YES!"

On the Move and Short on Time

I guarantee that there is a physical exercise for every lifestyle and schedule. Once you start doing your research, you will see I'm right as you come up with several possibilities. Make choices that will allow you to exercise regardless of the weather and that fit easily into the time you have available.

For example, let's say you found an exercise video on YouTube you enjoy. That's great, but don't stop there, check out more classes using the same search criteria as well as other classes with the same host. This variety will keep things interesting or even lead you to an abbreviated version of the workout you love so much that can be done when you're short on time.

Or perhaps you planned on taking a walk in the neighborhood but it rained. Don't let that stop you. Go to the local mall and walk indoors or repeatedly climb the stairs in your house for the same length of time. If you live in an apartment building, walk the halls or climb the stairs. Use your imagination.

The time to leave your excuses behind is here. Break down all your old barriers about exercise and commit to an exercise plan because exercise is what makes continued weight loss and weight maintenance not only doable, but also a reality!

How Often?

Exercise frequency has the greatest impact on weight loss. A well-regarded 2009 eight-week study on exercise frequency that is still respected today concluded that participants in all age groups who exercised four or more times per week achieved the greatest body fat loss, an average of 13.3 pounds.[19] Those who exercised less frequently experienced less weight loss, about four pounds each.

▶ *Exercise, improving weight and body composition can be done at any age (You are never too old, or too young).*

▶ *Building muscle is possible well into our eighties.*

▶ *Staying active is important for the mind as well as the body. Exercise reduces the risk of age-related dementia, Alzheimer's disease, and memory loss.*

▶ *Keeping the body moving has benefits beyond weight loss.*

▶ *Exercising helps you feel better, look better, think clearer, and puts you in a better mood.*

How can you pass all this up?

Lose Fat, Build Muscle

Another benefit of increased exercise is the increase in muscle mass which translates into a healthier, more toned body with a faster metabolism that burns more calories to increase weight loss and makes successful weight maintenance more likely. This is because muscle-building (strength-training) exercises increase and preserve metabolic rate. Muscle, being more metabolically active, burns more calories. Strength training is achieved by using free weights, including dumbbells, barbells, one's own body weight, and the weight-assisted machine common in gyms. If you've never lifted weights before, make sure to start with lifting light weights and getting some instruction.

An easy way to start lifting is to use cans of soup as weights (which weigh one pound) before progressing to something heavier. You can also use your body weight alone to build strength by performing pushups against a wall before progressing to doing them on the floor, which is more difficult.

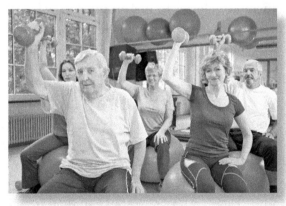

No matter what type of muscle-building exercise you choose, remember that they are done in two or three sets of 10-12 repetitions with a rest period between each set. A real time saver is to incorporate intervals of cardio during these "rest periods" thereby achieving two goals with one work out. Once again, check out all of the resources mentioned for finding cardio classes and instructional videos for safe muscle building.

Now, what you'll find out—perhaps unexpectedly—is that along with the perks that come from getting fit is the annoying fact that muscle weighs more than fat. This means that as you burn fat and build muscle you may not see huge results in the numbers on the scale—at least at first. That will change if you stick with your exercise program. Eventually you'll have proof in the scale that the pounds are decreasing as your body burns more calories faster. Even though muscle seems to weigh more than fat (a pound of muscle and a pound of fat are equally one pound), muscle burns fat more efficiently, makes you stronger, and has the added benefit of taking up less space (which you'll see in your clothes). For all these reasons, it's important that you make time to exercise.

Exercise Is Not a Ticket to Overeat

And last, but certainly not least, don't fool yourself into thinking that an increase in physical activity gives you permission to eat more calories! It's true that some people (usually athletes) need to increase calories to fuel an intense or lengthy period of exercise. However, additional calorie needs should be anticipated, and a plan formulated to spread them throughout the day to maintain satiety or whether or not to be eaten before or after workouts.

If you have any questions about the number of calories you should be eating, consult a registered dietitian. But for our purposes right now, I am discouraging high-calorie mocha coffee drink and muffins after the workout at the gym. It may just be to treat yourself, but do you really need three hundred or more extra calories snacks because you are feeling entitled after a workout? These "I was so good I can treat myself" feelings only serve one purpose and that is to add back any body fat burned in that exercise session, and sometimes even more.

It is also human nature to overestimate the number of calories burned throughout the day and during workouts. Even activity trackers have been found to be inaccurate in this regard as

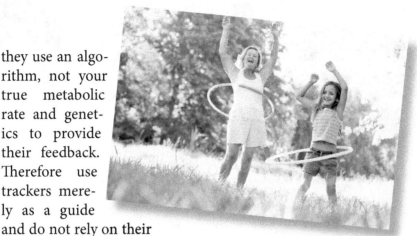

they use an algorithm, not your true metabolic rate and genetics to provide their feedback. Therefore use trackers merely as a guide and do not rely on their findings as gospel. Being unrealistic about the number of calories burned in a workout creates a calorie surplus. That's why you need to be aware of the fact that you must spend an average of 33.6 minutes on an elliptical trainer to burn the same number of calories contained in that fifty-gram energy bar you ate on your way to the gym. Or that it takes one hour of walking at a moderate pace to burn off the 250-calorie chocolate bar you ate last night while sitting on the couch watching TV. This makes it more logical to place the treadmill in front of the TV, doesn't it? It also goes without saying that any exercise equipment should, obviously, be seen as a food-free zone. My point is for you to be realistic about the number of calories you actually burn so you know that a light workout will never ever be able to compensate for eating a calorie-laden snack or large dessert. Remember the basics: When you don't burn off more calories than you eat you will have a calorie surplus and a calorie surplus *will* pack on pounds.

When it comes to losing weight it's commitment—not knowledge—that is power. When you commit and make the choice to change you'll lose weight. It's that simple. On the other hand, simply knowing will never get you to your goal unless you use that knowledge to say "I will" and then act on that commitment. Because where there is an "I will" there is a way.

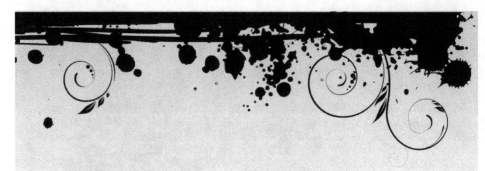

Your Goals for This Week:

1. Identify your social stumbling blocks and make an effort to overcome them

2. Practice your planned verbal responses to eating underminers, food pushers, and exercise bashers

3. Increase the frequency, duration, or intensity of your exercise routine to get more benefits from exercising

4. Build muscle and burn more calories by challenging your body by adding a new activity, sport, or exercise plan

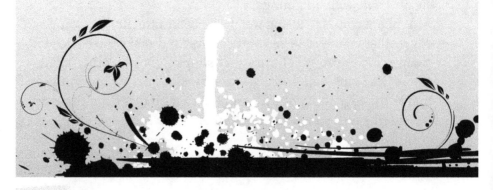

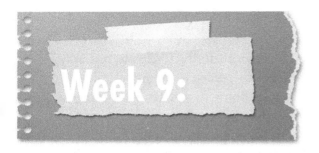

Attitude Adjustments

Thoughts and feelings both drive behavior, but it's our thoughts that determine how we feel about ourselves which in turn affects mood, how we interact with others, and, ultimately, if we succeed in any task. Our thoughts are also responsible for creating that internal dialogue we have with ourselves that is responsible for making us feel either good or lousy. The attitude we project based on these feelings affects how we interpret success.

The Power of Projecting a Positive Attitude

I want you to read the following two phrases out loud: "I lost another pound" and "I only lost a pound". Say them with the same intonation you would normally use when talking to yourself. Repeat them if you want because I need you to really hear yourself and take notice of how hearing each of these statements makes you feel. The purpose of this exercise is to show how the first statement definitely projects a positive attitude while the second is decidedly a negative one. Like the other tools you've learned, this one will also take practice to become a good habit.

To help you maintain a positive attitude, it helps to not only learn to catch yourself when you revert to negative talk, but to ask people you trust to also point it out. It's important to eliminate negative talk from your life because it leads to negative thoughts which leads to sabotaging your efforts, whereas positive talk leads to increasing short-term efforts which turns into long-term success. This is true for all aspects of your life but is especially true where weight loss and weight maintenance are concerned. Your every positive thought or action validates short-term success, therefore, it's so important to acknowledge every one of these successes.

If you need help staying positive, refer to the behavior chain in Chapter 5 before rereading the above statements. The behavior chain was designed to help you identify the consequence of a particular food behavior, particularly when thoughts about a poor food choice lead to feelings of guilt and shame. These emotions are powerful enough to overwhelm acceptance and block the mental energy to plan for next steps. If you did slip and overeat, don't panic. Instead think of what feeling bad and guilty about eating too much accomplishes besides triggering feelings of loss and futility. What a different outcome you would enjoy if you didn't feel so negative. Try to acknowledge your poor choice or indulgence and counteract it with a positive action such as exercising longer in the morning or compiling a shopping list of healthy foods to keep on hand. Your time is better spent searching the internet for a new project to keep from getting bored or learning to enjoy TV without being tempted by the food or candy commercials. Here are some ways you can make positive attitude adjustments.

Be Realistic

Setting realistic and attainable goals is the best thing you can do. Goals always need to be specific, doable, attainable, and measurable, so you can reach them and have a way to honestly assess and be able to celebrate your progress. The positive feelings and outcomes obtained by reaching a goal also allow for setting increasingly higher, but still reasonable, goals. This is what keeps the cycle of positive feelings going. So I caution you not to expect too much too fast, seek perfection, or let setbacks overwhelm you. Stay positive and learn from your mistakes.

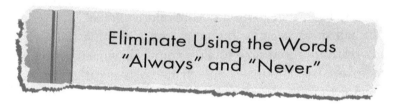

Eliminate Using the Words "Always" and "Never"

Making statements like "I will always exercise every day" or "I will never eat a cookie again" only burden you in ways that are counterproductive. To think that you will never miss a workout, or gain a couple of pounds, or not splurge at a BBQ is unrealistic and absurd. When you say never to any food, your desire for it will eventually increase to the point to where eating even a taste can trigger a binge which usually leads to feelings of failure. So, don't get caught in this trap and never say never because saying always and never only serves to weaken resolve to stick with any plan.

Substitute "More" for "Enough"

The question is not "Am I exercising enough?" but "Am I exercising more than I used to?" This book has consistently encouraged you to start from wherever you are and to challenge yourself to continually achieve more.

Your continued success is based on your continued efforts. Again, being able to interpret progress is based on setting and reaching realistic goals—which is what happens when you are consistently able to do more and more in all aspects of your life. Remember this when you successfully recover from setbacks by thinking positively about your new eating and exercise behaviors. Substitute questions that show you are always striving to improve, like, "Do I continue to get challenging physical activity?" "Do I continue to monitor my calorie intake?"

In banishing negative thoughts, you will think more clearly and creatively about how to alter your behavior to get back on your plan. This eliminates any chance of a negative emotional response to unmet expectations, food choices, food behaviors, and physical activity opportunities.

Don't Let the Bumps in the Road Slow You Down

Use those inevitable bumps in the road you will encounter on the road to your ultimate weight-loss success as opportunities to learn and refine the skills you'll need to reach your goals. Once again, success is based on trial and correction, not trial and error. Think of your weight-loss journey as a game and if the strategy you chose occasionally caused you to lose to another player, would that mean you would never play that game again? Of course not. Like playing a game, you'd try again by reshuffling the deck or rearranging the playing pieces or using a different strategy. Nothing in life goes smoothly and your path to a healthier weight is no different, so anticipate those bumps and be ready to smooth them by focusing on positive behaviors by acknowledging your accomplishments and your good choices. You will feel each of those bumps and some may slow you down, but they won't stop you cold. The momentary time outs they may cause will give you time to rethink the positive aspects of your journey. This is the chance to renew your focus in ways that lead to the positive emotional response you will need to continue on. For example, saying "I walked a lot on vacation even though I couldn't get to the gym, but I'll start going back to the gym this week" or "I know the scale is not always going to show a loss, especially when my salt intake affects water retention, so I will diligently record my food intake this week and avoid high-sodium foods." Or "It is unrealistic to follow my calorie goal every single day, but I really enjoyed the BBQ enough that I can live with the fact it will take a little longer to lose another two pounds. Maybe I'll exercise more to burn the extra calories."

The best strategy to recover from a setback begins with relying on past successes by recognizing and giving yourself credit for those times when you did your best, and to acknowledge

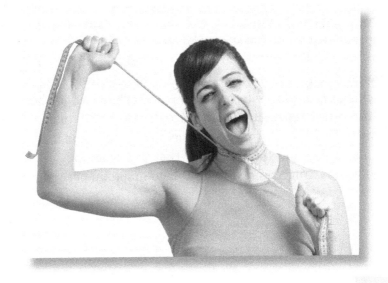

the circumstances that were particularly challenging. Then also assess the behaviors and skills you used to navigate those situations. Don't be afraid to also identify those instances when you could have done things differently or perhaps tried harder. Review each of these situations and you'll learn what you need to prepare for the next time a similar challenge arises. It will be your "AHA" moment.

Some of the "AHA" moments my clients have experienced come from focusing on their past positive successes. I remember one woman who was in week two of the program when she was invited to a christening where the food choices were all high-fat and high-carbohydrate, all choices that didn't fit into the food behaviors she had been practicing. Her strategy was to snack on a few bites of the least offensive food, enough to curtail her hunger until she got home to prepare a more appropriate dinner. Most important was that she felt great about how she had thought through her plan and executed it. This empowered her by proving that she was indeed able to stick to her new behaviors. The subject of her weight loss never entered into our exchange. She felt successful because of her behavior choice regardless of what she saw on the scale.

I had another client who had struggled with losing the same five pounds for months. Her daily food intake and exercise were appropriate except that she ate larger quantities of higher-calorie foods when she and her husband went out to dinner. Her "AHA" moment came when she realized she was not trying her best in sticking to her plan when eating out and acknowledged her need to do better. Her solution was to arm herself with a plan to order a low-fat salad or shrimp cocktail as an appetizer and to be aware of and follow her fullness cues. That was when her eating-out behaviors changed and she was able to maintain her weight.

Mirror, Mirror on the Wall

Too many of us define ourselves by size or body shape and that is alarming because it shifts the focus from health to weight as a standard or an ideal. Not only is this dangerous it also helps to encourage the growing incidence of body issues for everyone, no matter what their age. The media bears much of the responsibility for this as they publish heavily retouched photos of individuals with perfect skin and bodies or attractive actors, rail-thin models, and muscular hunks. Unfortunately, many who compare themselves to those beautiful people in the photos fail to realize that they probably have personal trainers and chefs and are paid to spend time on their appearance and body shape. Still others compare themselves to those around them, intensified by

social media. All of these comparisons too often lead to self-deprecation and poor body image. If you are tempted to compare your body to someone else's—don't. You have no idea of their genetic makeup or lifestyle. Or whether or not they've had cosmetic surgery. Or if they are thin due to an eating disorder or illness. If their body type is the best thing you like about them, you are defining their worth by their weight. That mode of thinking minimizes their positive qualities and negates yours. But what

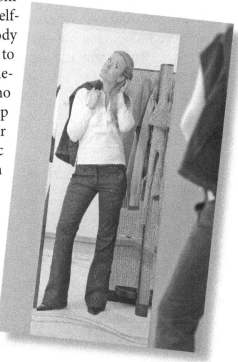

about what you cannot see? Are these people friendly, interesting, successful, and good to their friends, family, and community? We are so much more than what the scale tells us, so resist the urge to compare based on appearance.

Then there is the other side of the coin—society's stigma toward overweight individuals. Maybe you know how it feels to shop in a Big and Tall Shop or plus-size store. Why is it that being overweight says overindulgent or slovenly to some people? I have encountered people who were overweight because of a lack of nutrition education and those who were overweight as a result of the environment in which they lived. Some people have weight issues due to a medical condition or pharmacological therapy. In my personal experience, not one appeared overindulgent or had no regard for their personal appearance.

Self-esteem is often inflluenced by the number on the scale. But, again, to get back to my original point, how you look is not who you are. A negative body image sabotages any positive feelings you could be celebrating about any weight loss and improved health. Having a negative body image sets a person up for failure. That is why it is important to celebrate successes as an antidote for negative self-talk. Changing your body image is easy in theory, but not so easy to do. But it can be done. Like all the other behavior changes, it starts small, often by choosing one or two suggestions and practicing each one until they become a habit, before choosing one or two more. Practice these suggestions at every opportunity because having positive feelings about yourself is fundamental to your overall well-being—it gives you inner strength.

Change Your Body Image

"Accept the things you cannot change" is a line in several affirmations and a powerful statement that relates to overcoming many obstacles in life. In terms of weight loss, trying to lose those last five pounds is like trying to roll a boulder to the top of a mountain, one slip and it rolls right back to the bottom. Of course you should try your best to succeed, but if you have taken every step and can't lose those last pounds, maybe it means you are not ready or your body chemistry is working against you by determining you are at your comfortable weight. Instead of feeling bad consider your successes, work on being at the peak of wellness at any weight and enjoy your life.

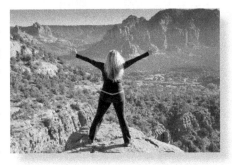

Celebrate your individuality. People come in different shapes and sizes; it is what makes us interesting. I remember my sister waiting until she was old enough to surgically remove a mole on her cheek just above her mouth. That mole made her feel like wearing a bag over her head. It bothered her so much. She was so relieved when it was removed, but, shortly after, Cindy Crawford became a supermodel and her face was

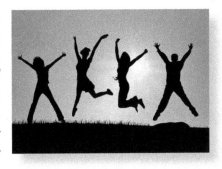

on every magazine cover sporting a very similar mark on her face. That made my sister miss the mole she had thought so long about removing because it was then that she realized it had made her face look interesting. Now, if we are able to enjoy different movies, books, professions, why can't we also celebrate different body shapes?

Appreciate what your body can do. We all have our strengths and abilities, be it practicing yoga, being a firefighter, or playing a great game of golf. When your body performs for you, you should be thankful. I had a poor body-image moment to overcome several months after the birth of my first child. Although I had 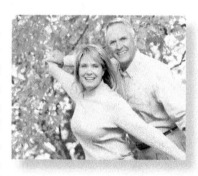 lost most of my baby weight, my body shape had changed. Every time I looked in the mirror, I felt disheartened. And then one day while looking in the mirror, I was overcome by wonder and gratitude for this body that had nurtured and given birth to a beautiful healthy baby. I vowed never to let myself bash it again.

Use positive outcomes to overcome negative experiences. I have counseled clients who avoided social situations that made them uncomfortable. One individual had not participated in a reunion of friends for years.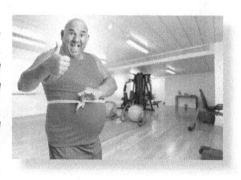

Another would not attend her spouse's business functions. But once they each acknowledged their efforts at behavior change and started celebrating successes of improved health, they no longer felt their weight was their most important attribute.

Find ways to reward yourself. It would be great if we all were surrounded by people who were full of compliments and an endless string of pats on the back, but we're not. It falls to all of us to be responsible for keeping up our own spirits. After all, each of us knows what we are capable of and how special we really are. Celebrate yourself.

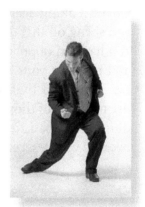

Dieting vs. Real Life

Living by any restrictive diet neither supports having a good body image nor empowers you. Trying to follow food rules that don't mesh with your food preferences or lifestyle is stressful. The media would like you to believe that one diet fits all or that fad diets work and that if a diet doesn't work for you, you did not do it right. We humans look for the easy way when it comes to dropping weight. Did anyone ever tell you that they lost twenty pounds and kept it off for the past five years, and that it wasn't hard? It's not simply eating low-fat, low-carb, etc., that leads to permanent weight loss. It's living in a healthy environment, practicing healthy eating habits, and continually making mindful choices in every situation that leads to a favorable outcome. Life is not a diet. Sometimes the low-fat cheese will work well on your sandwich and sometimes only the full-fat variety will work on the crackers. Sometimes the apple and almonds are an appropriate snack and sometimes eating an ice cream cone with your grandchild just makes your day. In living with your new plan, you will be making decisions like this all day, every day. So the sooner you shrug off that diet mentality, the sooner you will realize that you have an opportunity every three or four hours to try again and improve your intake or your exercise. Learn to enjoy that ice cream and then maybe suggest a trip to the playground to use up some of those calories or rethink what you are having for dinner or be satisfied that you had a successful guilt-free splurge because you deserved it.

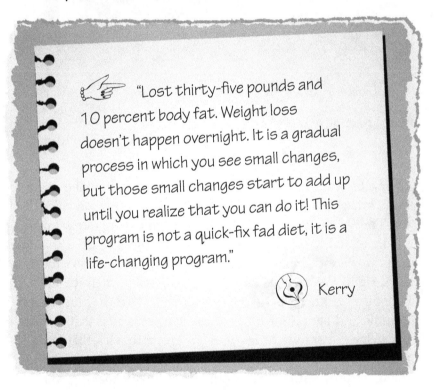

"Lost thirty-five pounds and 10 percent body fat. Weight loss doesn't happen overnight. It is a gradual process in which you see small changes, but those small changes start to add up until you realize that you can do it! This program is not a quick-fix fad diet, it is a life-changing program."

Kerry

Practice Intuitive Eating

The rigidity of a diet doesn't allow for common sense, practicality, or variation in lifestyles. Sure one afternoon snack is enough except when dinner is going to be late, then a second afternoon snack might be the answer if you skip the evening snack because chances are you won't be hungry before bedtime if you ate late.

The stress and fatigue attributed to dieting makes you more vulnerable to other life stresses. For some people, diets set up a never-ending cycle of stress and fatigue causing an increase in food intake followed by a diet that causes stress and fatigue. Sounds counterproductive to me.

Restrictive dieting doesn't allow people to follow hunger and fullness cues as it does not allow for intuitive eating. Intuitive eating, a type of mindful eating, was first described in 1995 by Evelyn Tribole and Elyse Resch, as having an awareness of what you are eating, how much you are eating, and why you are eating. Intuitive eating runs counter to a dieter's mentality by emphasizing that there is no right or wrong way to eat. Intuitive eaters make healthy food decisions, so even a food that is perceived as unhealthy or high calorie has less of an impact on weight and wellness when eaten in controlled portions.

To practice intuitive eating, ask yourself the following three questions before putting any food into your mouth:

1. *Am I hungry?* If the answer is no, don't eat. Maybe a non-food activity is what you need to entertain away the boredom or soothe your mood. If the answer is yes, read on.

2. *What am I hungry for?* This is your opportunity to decide for yourself what you want to eat. Without diet rules, it is your choice as to what food will satisfy your hunger.

3. *Did I make a good choice as to food and portion size?* Sure the fruit and nut snack might have been more nutritious, but

if the chips and guacamole are what you think will be most satisfying then grab the bowl and measuring spoon and have at it.

Many people follow diets without concern for eating balanced meals. Remember what I said about a healthy body losing and maintaining weight better. And how can you be happy if don't really enjoy what you are eating. Even people with diabetes or heart disease can eat French fries and ice cream when they are integrated in a way that is compatible with their meal plan. I can pretty much guarantee that the next best-selling fad diet will not show how to do that. However, you now have knowledge of the behaviors needed to form good habits and the decision-making guidelines to use to enjoy life and be successful in your health goals.

Stress: How it Affects Your Body

Following a plan should address your needs and reduce the uncertainty or restrictive cloud you have been living under. But there are other stresses that affect the way we eat.[20] The body responds to stress by what is called a fight-or-flight reaction. Emotional stress causes the same chemical changes in our body systems as coming face-to-face with a bear while walking in the woods. This is also much like the physiological changes you experience just after a near-miss car accident or the dread you feel when the phone rings after midnight. This feeling is caused, in part, by an increase in cortisol, the hormone your body needs to fight or run. Cortisol causes an increase in blood sugar and later a subsequent increased hunger. Cortisol increases anxiety and energy levels thereby burning more calories. This is what drives us to eat high-fat, high-calorie food to fuel the body's response to stress. During periods of long-term stress, however, these excess calories are not used but are stored as abdominal fat.[21]

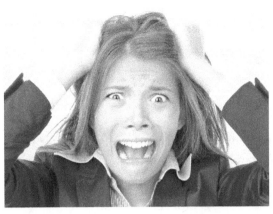

It is true that people eat more when they are stressed, while others lose their appetite. That response is often determined by whether the stress is sudden and acute, as in being fired or rushing to be with an ailing parent or child, or the ongoing stress of living with a teenager or having trouble paying your bills. It is not necessarily the amount or severity of the stress, but how one copes that determines the affect the stress has on food intake and weight. It is common for us to use food both to soothe and as a reward. Psychological distress causing emotional eating, binge eating, lower self-efficacy, and decreased self-esteem have been identified as significant predictors of weight loss and weight maintenance.[22] The key is to find more non-food ways to relieve stress. Relaxation techniques such as deep breathing and meditation are cited as two of the most powerful activities to de-stress.[23] Imagery, keeping a journal, yoga, dance, massage therapy, and music are also used to calm both the emotional and physical effects of stress.

Exercise: The Best Stress Reliever

My favorite stress-management technique is exercise because it not only keeps you on your path to weight loss and improved health, it also

- ▶ *raises endorphins, the "happy" brain chemicals*

- ▶ *improves mood*

- ▶ *reduces anxiety, increasing calm if performed on an ongoing basis*

- ▶ *promotes quality of sleep, decreasing fatigue*

- ▶ *soothes tense muscles*

- ▶ *improves physical well-being which then in turn improves mental health*

The next time you feel under stress may be the best time to get involved in any type of activity that works for you to counteract stress levels. Honestly, if it keeps you out of the pantry, the best activity may even be cleaning a closet or chopping wood. Whatever exercise you choose to do is good. Get moving and get calm.

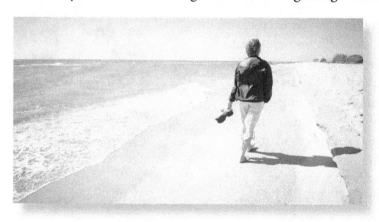

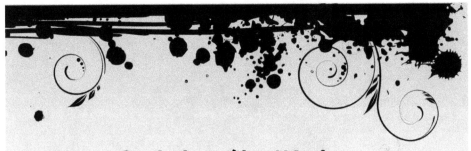

Your Goals for This Week:

1. Review your weight loss and health goals

   (You may need to revise them if you now think they originally were unrealistic.)

2. Work on removing words like "only", "never", "always", and "enough" from your vocabulary

3. Focus on the positive

   a. Acknowledge your accomplishments

4. Practice defining yourself by who you are and what you do and not by a number on the scale

5. Devise a plan to handle stress and replace stress eating with an activity

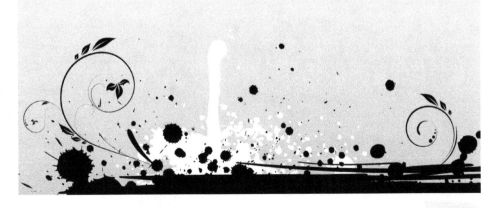

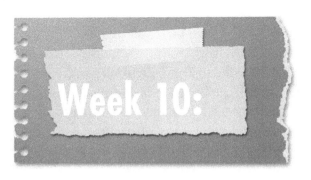

Mapping Your Future

You have reached the end of the beginning of your journey. You may not feel like you have arrived, but you now know where you are and that you're headed in the right direction. If you have reached the place you want to be health-wise and weight-wise, congratulations. If you are still on your way, it will now be easier to continue.

For some of you, the end of a weight loss program will be a positive experience with feelings of accomplishment and empowerment. For others, this ending brings with it a sense of dread because of the unknown of what happens next. "How will I continue to lose weight or keep the weight off?"

Maintaining Your Weight

For starters, no destructive self-talk. Saying things like "I am going to have trouble keeping the weight off" says it is time for an attitude adjustment and to formulate a constructive alternative. Your new attitude starts with saying "I am losing weight because of my new behavior changes and new skills.

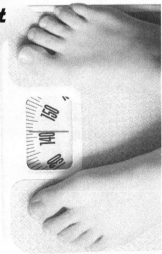

The program taught me what I needed to know. I will keep practicing my new habits." Instead of "The program is ending and I have so much more weight to lose," tell yourself "It took time to gain the weight, it is going to take time to lose. I have been losing weight. I will stick with the plan and maintain the behavior changes that made me healthy."[24]

This new internal dialogue is you being your very own cheering section. If you continue to imagine your weight loss effort as a journey, visualize the crowd that has lined your route and is now waiting for you at the finish line with words of encouragement and celebrations of success. Have you ever been to an event where the spectators were cheering "You can do it," "Way to go," or "Keep it going"? Well, the idea is to do the same for yourself.

It is great to have encouraging family and friends, but if your internal dialogue sends you negative messages, your negative thoughts will lead to negative effort, which diminishes the likelihood of short-term and, therefore, long-term success. So stay positive.

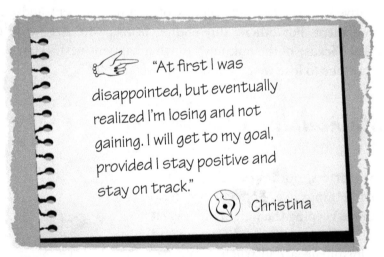

"At first I was disappointed, but eventually realized I'm losing and not gaining. I will get to my goal, provided I stay positive and stay on track."

Christina

This doesn't mean you stop accepting encouragement from family and friends. Social support and acknowledgment are important and essential for both self-esteem, continued motivation and many other reasons. The support of the people close to you makes it easier to ask for child-care help so you have time to exercise. It may also involve asking for and receiving help from a spouse or parent to help with food shopping and meal preparation. Help may also come from coworkers who can become more sensitive and not leave food where it can tempt you. Maybe your coworkers will also become more accepting of choosing restaurants for lunch with more appropriate menu options. Never be afraid to tell those around you what you need to be more successful or suggest ways they can help remove barriers to help you change (they can't read your mind). Enlisting help and being open to accepting that support only adds to your chances of success and increases acceptance of your behavior changes.

Sound Advice from Long-Term Weight Loss Maintainers

Never underestimate what you can learn from those who have lost significant weight and kept it off for a long time.

The National Weight Loss Registry tracks highly successful individuals and, interestingly, finds that they have no single method or diet plan in common—other than some form of calorie restriction. What they did have in common was how they kept the weight off. For example:

► *Eating a lower fat diet, 25-30% of total calories, despite the latest research finding that dietary fat is not the enemy in the battle of the bulge*

► *Counting calories and adhering to a daily calorie goal by eating portion-controlled, low-calorie dense foods*

► *Self-monitoring, keeping a food journal, for example*

- ► *Engaging in high levels of physical activity, especially planned exercise of approximately 60 minutes every day to boost metabolism*

- ► *Consistent behaviors, such as practicing healthy habits, sticking to mealtimes and exercise schedules*

- ► *Always eating breakfast*

- ► *Getting a good night's sleep*

- ► *Practicing mindful eating, through an awareness of how different foods affect feelings, thoughts, and physical sensations by paying attention to the temperature, texture, and taste when eating.*

By following these strategies you, too, will join these individuals who found the secret to long-term weight loss success

Create a Positive Social Environment

It stands to reason that some people are more successful at weight loss when they are members of a group with this same goal. There are many commercial weight-loss group programs that lend this type of support, but you can also create your own positive social environment. You need to start by sharing what you've learned with your family, friends, and coworkers. You may be surprised to find that they have seen the changes in you and wish to follow in your footsteps. Maybe by sharing your new food behaviors or inviting others to join you for your walks will not only help and support you, but also expresses an interest and signals that you care about helping someone close to you. The participants in my live programs often share with me that their spouse or another family member is following along with them and successfully losing weight. Creating the social environment that helps you thrive also provides that same opportunity for others. You can also take it a step further when the people around you actively show interest. If this is the case, consider forming a group that meets once a week to discuss the chapter in this book you are currently working on. This opens the door to swapping food and activity journals and critiquing each other. The constructive suggestions that come from this sharing will lead to many positive actions such as suggesting alternative menus and food choices, exercise plans, etc. You could even hold these meetings during walks thereby increasing your opportunity to exercise. This exchange of information increases accountability of everyone in the group (even you!) as well as is an opportunity to experiment with new ideas for success.

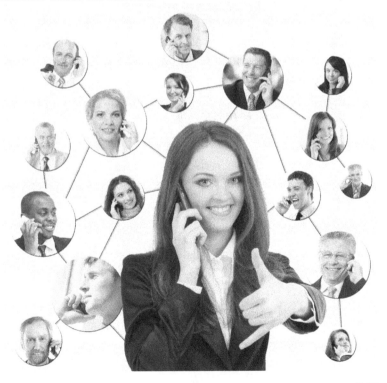

When the Weight Loss Stops

There will come a time when you will stop losing weight or even regain a few pounds. This is normal and it does not mean you have failed. It is also not a need for grave concern as the body is doing what it is biologically designed to do—sustain weight. Here's what happens: When you achieve a certain amount of weight loss you start fighting against body systems. Brain chemicals begin to fight to replace fat stores by increasing enzyme production to encourage fat storage, which makes maintaining lost weight not so easy.

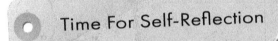

Time For Self-Reflection

If you have experienced this situation or if you noticed an increase in appetite, consider trying any of the following options that apply to you:

► *You may need to recalculate calorie needs to reduce food intake to a level more appropriate to your lower weight.*

► *You may need to increase your calorie intake to continue to lose weight if your diligence has caused you to under-eat your way into starvation mode and slowed the rate your body burns calories.*

► *You may need to adjust the frequency or duration of your exercise or choose a more challenging activity to increase calorie burn.*

► *You may no longer be eating the correct portion sizes, so double-check yourself and go back to measuring.*

> ▶ *You may need to start keeping a food journal which (chances are) you stopped when things were going well. It's common to hear that when people stop journaling they stop adhering to the plan because it took away their accountability.*

Even if in spite your best efforts your weight loss stops, you should consider it a victory because if you hadn't lost the weight in the first place you'd never have gotten to this next step—weight management. You now have the opportunity to allow your brain and body to adjust to your lower weight through the self-preservation mechanisms programmed in your DNA. These mechanisms keep your body within the weight range it is accustomed to—the set-point—which many people refer to as a plateau. But even though this is annoying, especially when you need to lose more weight for health reasons, a weight loss plateau gives the body and brain the opportunity to establish a new lower set-point to maintain. Even if you do not reach your goal weight, reaching a plateau means you have stopped gaining weight, so that's weight you won't have to lose again. So whether or not you managed to reach your goal weight you can consider yourself a success!

Reassess Your Motivation

This is the point at which you need to honestly assess your motivation and methods as carefully as you scrutinized them when you started the program outlined in this book. If you have successfully lost five, ten, or twenty pounds, then it makes sense to keep using these exact same tools and techniques until you reach your ultimate goal. If not, it means that you may need to start over from page 1. This often happens, so you aren't alone, and I know this because when I give this program to live audiences, I see familiar faces. This is not because my program doesn't work, it's because some people need more time to change a lifetime of not-so-healthy eating habits. Some people repeat the program immediately and some after a year or more. These individuals know they are free to join me whenever they need help. My only rules are that they attend every session, keep food logs, and continue to exercise at the appropriate level. I have designed my program with those criteria because that is what many people need to be successful. I am also committed to working for anyone as long as they work for themselves because the results are profound.

Now that you've gotten to the end of this book, chances are you have experienced weight loss, and you are now on your way to having long-term success in keeping it off. You are motivated to keep to the path that got you here successfully. You have learned how to balance your calories, navigate the menu and food requests when eating out, techniques for avoiding social sand traps, and ways to shop for and cook higher-quality food. You also know how to sidestep temptation, occasionally splurge, and how to get back on track when you need to. Best of all, you've also learned to celebrate milestones and it is my fervent wish that you enjoyed the journey.

"My body is fighting me for every inch and pound now after losing 18.2 pounds over the past three months. I am angry that the scale seems to have stopped showing a significant amount of weight loss in the past two weeks. Without your good advice, I would be trying to starve myself . . . and then eat a ton because

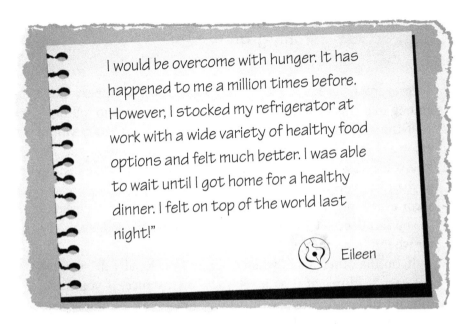

I would be overcome with hunger. It has happened to me a million times before. However, I stocked my refrigerator at work with a wide variety of healthy food options and felt much better. I was able to wait until I got home for a healthy dinner. I felt on top of the world last night!"

Eileen

Maintaining good health should never be a burden or a chore. Likewise, a workout should be enjoyed as "me" time, and cooking dinner for yourself or your family should always be an expression of caring and love.

Slip, Slide, Crash and Burn

If something goes wrong, as it almost assuredly will, how quickly you recover is important and that will depend on whether you're recovering from a slip, a slide, or a crash and burn.

► A slip is a one-time error in judgment or poor choice.

► A slide is made up of many slips over time or a return to former habits and behaviors.

► A crash and burn means there is little hope of recovery and the chance of returning to a positive and healthy lifestyle is slim.

Putting on the Brakes

To prevent a slip from becoming a slide down a slippery slope ending in a crash and burn, here are some strategies to follow:

If the slip was a mindful food choice, as in "I really would enjoy a donut." Or maybe it was a birthday celebration and before you realized it, you had eaten a whole slab of cake instead of the taste you had planned. When this happens, be sure you savor every morsel and make eating it a pleasurable experience so you feel completely satisfied and able to acknowledge this slip for what it is, a splurge.

If, on the other hand, when a slip is emotionally driven, it is not easy to think of it as a splurge. For instance, if you had a difficult day, and either with planned malice or mindless happenstance, you were already on the other end of the drive-thru with a cheeseburger and fries, a bag of cheese puffs, or a pint of ice cream when the guilt hit. In this case, you need to acknowledge the incident for what it was, an error in judgment. Admit to yourself that everyone makes mistakes, including you, and that to err is human. To think that you would never revert to a former behavior or an unhealthy food choice is unrealistic and absurd. So, forgive yourself. Guilt and regret are wasted emotions that misuse mental energy, keep you stuck in the moment, and prevent you from thinking about what is really important. In this case, what is important is to consider how to affect the outcome and reduce the likelihood of this type of incident happening again. Evaluate not only the emotional and social factors that precipitated making the poor decision, but also, the environment in which the slip occurred. If it was emotionally or socially driven, figure out what you could have changed and remember it the next time you are in that situation. Right now is the time to plan how to get back on track. (It may also be helpful to revisit the Behavior Chain exercise in week 5.)

I remember one client who discovered that she overate whenever she ate out with a certain group of friends, despite her new skills. After a number of slips, she suggested a change of venue for their get-togethers. Instead of eating, she suggested a movie or declined the invitation altogether until she honed her verbal skills to the point that she could avoid social sand traps.

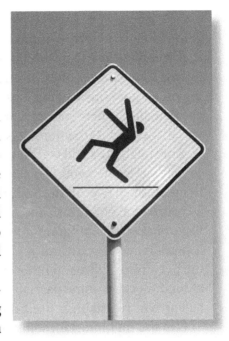

Another client was overwhelmed by the aroma coming from the bakery she passed on her way home from work. After working a particularly long day, those smells just sucked her in the door to buy a cinnamon roll or two. Her bakery pit stop was an emotionally and environmentally driven indulgent and not a well-thought-through decision. She rightly decided that this undermining of her weight-loss efforts required a different route home.

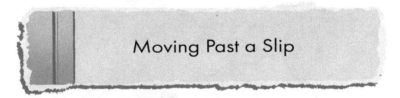

Moving Past a Slip

The best way to move forward after a slip is to simply leave it behind without diminishing your enjoyment. If that sundae or rack of ribs tasted good, acknowledge it. However, if you indulge in a food you have been depriving yourself of, this may be a wake-up call to figure out how you can work that food into your plan. Deprivation is one of the reasons for overeating. There are ways to eating your crave-worthy food more often without breaking gerously close to former unhealthy behaviors. Take this as a sign that you have lost focus and it is time for some hard work and introspection. Slides often mean a change in motivation or slacking off or stopping keeping logs and removing a source of being accountable. When you stop practicing healthy eating skills in social or stressful situations, it is very easy to return to old habits. If your weight loss and weight maintenance remain as important as they were when you first started this program, then it's easier to nip this behavior in the bud and put a stop to a slide and make a U-turn to avoid a crash and burn. Do this by going back to the beginning of this program if you need to. In the same way that it takes longer to drive to a place for the first time, starting at the beginning will not take as long for weight changes this time around. Because some parts of the route will be familiar, the behavior will re-establish itself quickly. Just don't skip any steps. This is also an important solution to remember when faced with any weight regain. Catch the trend early and retrace your steps or start from the beginning. It is much easier to lose three to five pounds of regained weight than ten to fifteen pounds if you wait too long.

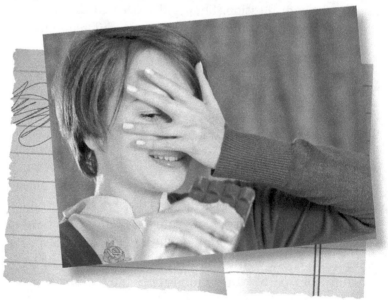

A former client recently returned for counseling when she regained the twenty pounds she lost three years prior. After three weeks of refresher courses, she is happily nine pounds lighter and once again empowered.

Reach Your Destination, Enjoy the Journey

Here are ways to navigate social situations, stress, travel, celebrations, and everyday life which all present obstacles to sustaining healthy eating habits. It takes mindfulness, effort, and planning to navigate and identify the detours and challenges before you can come up with a solution leading to making healthier choices.

Splurge and enjoy, a big meal, or occasionally have seconds of dessert without feeling guilty, deprived, or remorseful in order to enjoy every bite. If you don't fully enjoy the food experience, you will be left unfulfilled and wanting more.

Do the things that bring you joy. Now that you've established that it is necessary to exercise for health, find an activity that you enjoy so you'll look forward to doing it. Think back to what you used to do for fun. Dancing is often reminiscent of good times. Pickle ball is all the rage as it reminds people of the ball games of their youth. Walks either on park trails or on a beach in your town or neighborhood can also feel like a mini vacation.

Paving the Way To Successful Weight Loss

At the beginning of this program, I made you aware of the tremendous influence your environment has on when, where, what, and how much you eat. The environment bombards all our senses with cues that encourage us to eat and eat a lot. Also explained was how your psychological well-being, your past experiences, and your upbringing also influence why you eat at times of stress, celebration, and reward. You now have the skills to change your environment and your mind and the knowledge to continue to identify obstacles and inappropriate enticements as well as how you respond to them. You are on your way to providing yourself with an environment that nurtures healthy eating and exercise habits, including appropriate food availability, supportive family, friends, and coworkers, and opportunities for entertaining physical activity.

Whether your overall weight loss goal is five pounds or fifty, you now have the strategies for evaluating your food choices, portion sizes, and food behaviors that have been roadblocks on your weight loss journey. You can also identify the small changes that translate to incremental, specific, realistic, achievable, and measurable short-term goals. Over time, practicing these strategies helps them to become the habits that lead you to lose the weight and keep it off. Keep in mind, you can eat today for a healthier tomorrow.

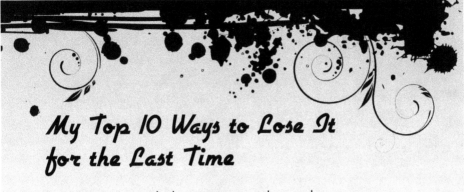

My Top 10 Ways to Lose It for the Last Time

1. Focus on your behaviors, not on the number you see on the scale

2. Begin every day with a balanced breakfast

3. Fill half your plate with vegetables and the rest with a combination of lean proteins, complex carbohydrates, and low-fat milk/yogurt products

4. Practice portion control

5. Plan to eat meals and snacks to avoid extreme hunger

6. Be aware of and follow hunger and satiety cues

7. Limit eating foods that are high in fat and sugar

8. Eat mindfully

9. Integrate physical activity into your daily routine

10. Think positively, respect your body, and nurture your spirit

You are ready to map your path to health and wellness. Enjoy the journey!

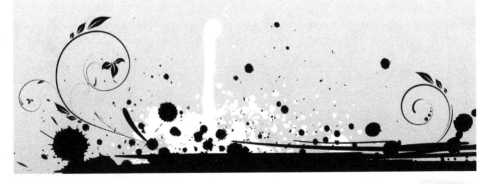

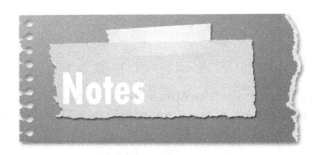

Notes

Week 1

1. Dorothy Van Buren, PhD, and Meghan M Sinton, PhD, "Psychological Aspects of Weight Loss and Weight Maintenance," *JADA* 109, no. 12, (December 2009): 1994–1996.

2. Anwar T. Merchant et al., "Carbohydrate Intake and Overweight and Obesity among Healthy Adults," *JADA* 109, no. 7, (July 2009): 1165–1172.

3. Frank M. Sacks, MD, et al., "Preventing Overweight Using Novel Dietary Strategies," *New England Journal of Medicine* 360, (Feb 2009): 859-873.

4. Jack Hollis, PhD, et al., Kaiser Permanente, July 8 2008; "Keeping a Food Diary Doubles Weight Loss," *American Journal of Preventative Medicine*, (August 2008).

5. W. C. Miller, D. M. Kyocera, and E. J. Hamilton, "A Meta-Analysis of the Past 25 Years of Weight Loss Research Using Diet, Exercise or Diet Plus Exercise Intervention," *International Journal of Obesity* 21, no. 10, (October 1997): 941–947.

Week 2

6. Paul S. MacLean et al., "Regular Exercise Attenuates the Metabolic Drive To Regain Weight After Long-Term Weight Loss," *American Journal Physiology-Regulatory, Integrative and Comparative Physiology* 297, (September 2009): R793–R802.

7. Levine, J. (2003). Non-exercise activity thermogenesis. *Proceedings of the Nutrition Society,* 62(3), 667-679. doi:10.1079/PNS2003281.

Week 3

8. St. Jeor Mifflin, MD, et al., "A New Predictive Equation for Resting Energy Expenditure in Healthy Individuals," *Journal of the American Dietetic Association* 51, (2005): 241–247.

9. Dorling, J. L., Van Vliet, S., Huffman, K. M., Kraus, W. E., Bhapkar, M., Pieper, C. F., ... & CALERIE Study Group. (2021). Effects of caloric restriction on human physiological, psychological, and behavioral outcomes: highlights from CALERIE phase 2. *Nutrition Reviews,* 79 (1), 98-113.

10. Fechner, E., Smeets, E. T., Schrauwen, P., & Mensink, R. P. (2020). The effects of different degrees of carbohydrate restriction and carbohydrate replacement on cardiometabolic risk markers in humans—a systematic review and meta-analysis. *Nutrients,* 12(4), 991.

11. Anwar T. Merchant, ScD, DMD, Hassanali Vatanparast, MD, PhD, et al., "Carbohydrate Intake and Overweight and Obesity among Healthy Adults," *JADA* 109, (2009): 1165–1172.

Week 4

12. Barbara Rolls, *The Volumetrics Eating Plan*, (New York: William Morrow Paperbacks, 2007).

Week 5

13. Jennifer Mathieu ,"What Should You Know about Mindful and Intuitive Eating?" *JADA* 109, issue 2, (2009): 1982–1987.

14. Brian Wansink, PhD, Junyong Kim, PhD, Dept. of Applied Economics and Mgmt., Cornell University, Ithaca, NY, "Bad Popcorn in Big Buckets: Portion Size Can Influence Intake as Much as Taste," *Journal of Nutrition Education and Behavior* 37, no. 5, (Sept-Oct): 242–245.

15. Brian Wansink, PhD, *Mindless Eating: Why We Eat More Than We Think*, (New York: Bantam Books, 2006).

Week 6

16. Beck, M. E. (2007). Dinner preparation in the modern United States. *British Food Journal.*

Week 7

17. Lorien E. Urban, MS, et al., "The Accuracy of Stated Energy Contents of Reduced-Energy, Commercially Prepared Foods," *JADA* 110, issue 1, (January 2010): 116–123.

Week 8

18. R. R.Wing and R. W. Jeffrey, "Benefits of Recruiting Participants with Friends and Increasing Social Support for Weight Loss and Weight Maintenance," *Journal of Consulting and Clinical Psychology* 67, no. 1, (1999):132–138.

19. F. B. Willis et al., "Frequency of Exercise for Body Fat Loss: A Controlled Cohort Study," *Journal of Strength and Conditioning Research* 23, no. 8, (Nov 2009): 2377–2380.

Week 9

20. https://www.enprc.emory.edu/about/news/developmental_cognitive_neuroscience/stress_overeating.html

21. Mary F. Dallman, Norman Pecoraro et al., "Chronic Stress and Obesity: A New View of 'Comfort Food,'" http://www.pnas.org/cgi/doi/10.1073/pnas.1934666100, *PNAS* 100, no. 20, (Sept 30, 2003): 11697–11701.

22. Dorothy Van Buren, PhD, and Meghan M Sinton, PhD, "Psychological Aspects of Weight Loss and Weight Maintenance," *JADA* 109, no. 12, (December 2009): 1994–1996.

23. Gian Mauro Mazoni, PsyD, et al., "Can Relaxation Training Reduce Emotional Eating in Women with Obesity? An Exploration Study with 3 Months of Follow-up," *Journal of the American Dietetic Association* 109, (2009): 1427–1432.

Week 10

24. Kelly D. Brownell, PhD, The LEARN Program For Weight Management.

The Well-Stocked Kitchen

Beyond Sugar, Flour, Salt, and Pepper

The Well-Stocked Refrigerator

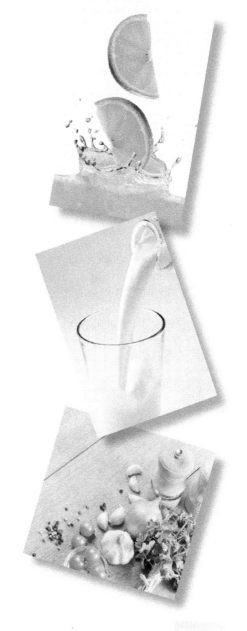

Jarred minced garlic

Dijon mustard

Low–sodium soy sauce

Low–sodium ketchup

Worcestershire sauce

Fat–free Italian dressing

Maple syrup

Orange juice

Lemon juice

Low–fat or nonfat milk

Nonfat yogurt

Eggs

Egg substitute

Fat–free margarine

Parmesan cheese

Low–fat cheese

Fat–free cream cheese

Refrigerator (con't.)

Butter

Shredded part–skim mozzarella

Lemons

Limes

Onions

Shallots

Potatoes

Jarred pesto

Fat–free margarine

Fat–free sour cream

Fat–free plain yogurt

Reduced–fat mayo

Lettuce

Tomatoes

Cucumbers

Carrots

Fresh fruit

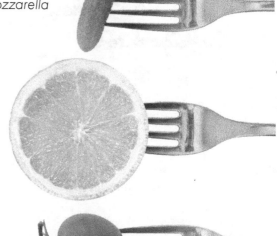

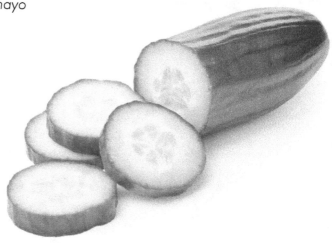

The Well-Stocked Cabinet

Olive oil

Canola oil

Cooking spray

Balsamic vinegar

Cider vinegar

White vinegar

Rice vinegar

Garlic powder

Dried rosemary

Dried oregano

Dried thyme

Dried tarragon

Dried basil

Dried dill

Ground ginger

Crushed red pepper

Bread crumbs

Honey

Sesame seeds

Tabasco

Sugar

Corn starch

Flour

Brown sugar

Peanut butter

Canned tomatoes
(15-ounce and 28-ounce)

Tomato sauce

Tomato paste

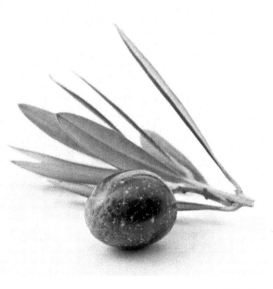

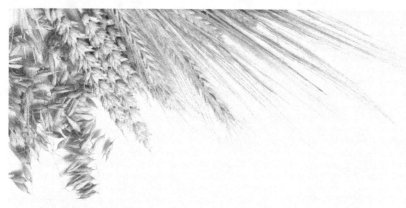

Cabinet (con't.)

Low–sodium vegetable broth

Low–sodium chicken broth

Pasta

Rice, white and brown

Canned beans, red kidney,
  cannellini, chick peas

Dried cranberries

Dried apricots

Raisins

Raspberry preserves

Apricot preserves

Bran cereal

Whole wheat bread

White wine

Red wine

Cooking sherry

Walnuts, whole
  and chopped

Almonds, whole
  and slivered

Canned tuna (in water)

The Well-Stocked Freezer

Frozen cooked shrimp

Frozen boneless chicken breasts

Frozen fish filets

Frozen vegetables, i.e. spinach, green beans, peas, broccoli

Orange juice concentrate

Sliced whole grain bread

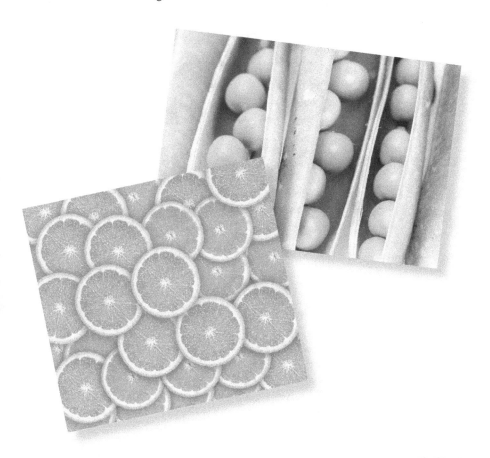

Chapter 2

Color Symphony/Shutterstock.com
Action Sports Photography/Shutterstock.com
Rafal Olkis/Shutterstock.com
Lukiyanova Natalia/frenta/Shutterstock.com
Stuart Jenner/Shutterstock.com
Worytko Pawel/Shutterstock.com
ollyy/Shutterstock.com

Chapter 3

leoks/Shutterstock.com
idea for life/Shutterstock.com
MimagePhotography/Shutterstock.com
Olaf Speier/Shutterstock.com
studiogi/Shutterstock.com
Yellowj/Shutterstock.com
spotmatik/Shutterstock.com
Subbotina Anna/Shutterstock.com
Sergej Nivens/Shutterstock.com
donatas 1205/Shutterstock.com

Chapter 4

Kokhanchikov/Shutterstock.com
Asier Romero/Shutterstock.com
fotogiunta/Shutterstock.com
aboikis/Shutterstock.com
Ekaterina Nikitina/Shutterstock.com
Stephen VanHorn/Shutterstock.com
XAOC/Shutterstock.com
Maceofoto/Shutterstock.com
Chepko Danil Vitalevich/Shutterstock.com
Tomo Jessenicnik/Shutterstock.com
vesna cvorovic/Shutterstock.com
Sandra Caldwell/Shutterstock.com
Antonio Jorge Nunes/Shutterstock.com
Beata Becia/Shutterstock.com
AMA/Shutterstock.com
photobank.kiev.ua/Shutterstock.com

Chapter 5

AlexAnnaButs/Shutterstock.com
Picsfive/Shutterstock.com
Fotocrisis/Shutterstock.com
Michael C. Gray/Shutterstock.com
Billy Wolf/Shutterstock.com
freesoulproduction/Shutterstock.com
Alex Staroseltsev/Shutterstock.com
ktsDesign/Shutterstock.com
omkar.a.v/Shutterstock.com
Andy Dean Photography/Shutterstock.com

Chapter 6

L.M.V./Shutterstock.com
pzAxe/Shutterstock.com
Monkey Business Images/Shutterstock.com
Hannamariah/Shutterstock.com
wavebreak media/Shutterstock.com
Tyler Olson/Shutterstock.com
Subbotina Anna/Shutterstock.com
Olena Mykhaylova/Shutterstock.com
Yuri Arcurs/Shutterstock.com
AlessandroBiasciolo/Shutterstock.com

Chapter 7

L.M.V./Shutterstock.com
Blend Images/Shutterstock.com
leoks/Shutterstock.com
Christi Tolbert/Shutterstock.com
Nejron Photo/Shutterstock.com

Chapter 8

Quintanilla/Shutterstock.com
Roma Koshel/Shutterstock.com
EpicStockMedia/Shutterstock.com
Piotr Marcinski/Shutterstock.com
kavring/Shutterstock.com
Robert Kneschke/Shutterstock.com
Monkey Business Images/Shutterstock.com

Chapter 9

Dirima/Shutterstock.com
Miodrag Trajkovic/Shutterstock.com
srecko80/Shutterstock.com
Deborah Kolb/Shutterstock.com
kurhan/Shutterstock.com
Luis Louro/Shutterstock.com
jayfish/Shutterstock.com
Maridav/Shutterstock.com
Piotr Marcinski/Shutterstock.com
Yarygin/Shutterstock.com

Chapter 10

cosma/Shutterstock.com
EDHAR/Shutterstock.com
Jarrod Boord/Shutterstock.com
Aletia/Shutterstock.com
iofoto/Shutterstock.com
Warren Goldswain/Shutterstock.com

Back Matter

Olena Mykhaylova/Shutterstock.com
Olga Lyubkina/Shutterstock.com
Chepko Danil Vitalevich/Shutterstock.com
vesna cvorovic/Shutterstock.com
Anna Sedneva/Shutterstock.com
Maceofoto/Shutterstock.com
Beata Becia/Shutterstock.com
Hofhauser/Shutterstock.com
Fotocrisis/Shutterstock.com

CPSIA information can be obtained
at www.ICGtesting.com
Printed in the USA
JSHW031929300123
36995JS00002B/38